Myopathies in Clinical Practice

Myopathies

in Clinical Practice

Edited by

Phillip R J Barnes PhD FRCP
Consultant Neurologist, King's College Hospital, London, UK

David Hilton-Jones MD FRCPE FRCP
Consultant Neurologist, Radcliffe Infirmary, Oxford, UK

With contributions from

Marinos C Dalakas MD
Chief, Neuromuscular Disease Section, NINDS, National Institutes of Health, Bethesda, MD, USA

Jacqueline A Palace MD FRCP
Consultant Neurologist, Radcliffe Infirmary, Oxford, UK

Michael R Rose MD FRCP
Consultant Neurologist, King's College Hospital, London, UK

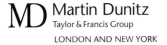
MD Martin Dunitz
Taylor & Francis Group
LONDON AND NEW YORK

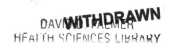

© 2003 Martin Dunitz, an imprint of the Taylor & Francis Group

First published in the United Kingdom in 2003
by Martin Dunitz, an imprint of the Taylor & Francis Group,
11 New Fetter Lane, London EC4P 4EE

Tel.:   +44 (0) 20 7583 9855
Fax.:   +44 (0) 20 7842 2298
E-mail: info@dunitz.co.uk
Website: http://www.dunitz.co.uk

A CIP record for this book is available from the British Library.

ISBN 1 899066 71 3

Distributed in the USA by
Fulfilment Center
Taylor & Francis
10650 Tobben Drive
Independence, KY 41051, USA
Toll Free Tel.: +1 800 634 7064
E-mail: taylorandfrancis@thomsonlearning.com

Distributed in Canada by
Taylor & Francis
74 Rolark Drive
Scarborough, Ontario M1R 4G2, Canada
Toll Free Tel.: +1 877 226 2237
E-mail: tal_fran@istar.ca

Distributed in the rest of the world by
Thomson Publishing Services
Cheriton House
North Way
Andover, Hampshire SP10 5BE, UK
Tel.: +44 (0)1264 332424
E-mail: salesorder.tandf@thomsonpublishingservices.co.uk

Composition by Scribe Design, Gillingham, Kent, UK

Printed and bound in Spain by Grafos SA.

Contents

Contributors

Phillip R J Barnes PhD FRCP
Consultant Neurologist
King's College Hospital
London
UK

Marinos C Dalakas MD
Chief
Neuromuscular Diseases Section
NINDS
National Institutes of Health
Bethesda
MD
USA

David Hilton-Jones MD FRCPE FRCP
Consultant Neurologist
Radcliffe Infirmary
Oxford
UK

Jacqueline A Palace MD FRCP
Consultant Neurologist
Radcliffe Infirmary
Oxford
UK

Michael R Rose MD FRCP
Consultant Neurologist
King's College Hospital
London
UK

Preface

Although symptoms relating to the muscles such as myalgia, fatigue and cramps are extremely common, most of the myopathies are very rare indeed. It is therefore difficult for a clinician with an average practice to gain much experience in the recognition of different types of muscle disease, let alone their optimum management.

The clinical care of patients with myopathies is also a meeting point for a number of medical specialities. Neurologists, rheumatologists and paediatricians, together with some orthopaedic surgeons feel that the myopathies rightly belong to them. All bring a different approach to diagnosis and management but need to acquire some of the skills of the other specialities if they are to provide the best care for their patients. The skills of other disciplines, the therapists, nurses and even social workers are also very important if we are to rise to the challenge of providing truly responsive multidisciplinary care.

The myopathies are also amongst the most fascinating group of disorders both to treat and to study. Much of the cutting edge of the 'new genetics' was performed in the study of muscle disease. Also, much of the work that remains to be done in terms of treatment of genetic diseases will be pioneered in patients with muscle diseases. We hope that some of our enthusiasm for this group of diseases will be conveyed to our readers.

There are many larger books on the subject which are excellent but probably beyond the requirements of a 'jobbing' neurologist or rheumatologist. The general neurology and rheumatology books tend to provide very little information and may confuse the reader. Our goal is to provide the general clinician with a practical manual for their encounters with myopathies. We have biased the content towards clinical assessment and towards those disorders which are commonest, or of particular importance. We have tried to be as up to date as possible with genetic and other advances but in such a fast moving field it is inevitable that those aspects of this volume will age faster than the rest.

Phillip R J Barnes & David Hilton-Jones

Acknowledgements

No neuromuscular service can function without the support of many colleagues in many fields. Special mention, however, must be made of the excellent help we receive from our histopathology colleagues. Dr Waney Squier in Oxford, and Drs Safa Al-Sarraj and Susan Robinson at King's provide us with an excellent diagnostic service and have kindly allowed us to use much of their histological material in this book.

We thank also our respective spouses and children for love and forbearance, the publishers for their patience and our patients for their friendship.

BASIC PRINCIPLES

chapter 1

Clinical assessment

In much of clinical practice a secure diagnosis can be achieved on the basis of clinical evaluation alone. That is, by history taking and physical examination, without resort to specific investigative techniques. In the field of muscle diseases (myopathies) there are only a few disorders (Table 1.1) that are so characteristic that they can be diagnosed with relative certainty at the bedside. However, this does not detract from the importance of careful clinical evaluation, for the information so obtained is very likely to indicate the nature of the problem, even if not the specific diagnosis. The clinical features may suggest that the problem is most likely to be a dystrophy, or inflammatory myopathy, or metabolic disorder, etc, and this deduction will be of considerable help in deciding upon the order of subsequent investigations. A blunderbuss approach to the laboratory assessment of a patient complaining of weakness may at worst prove fruitless, or at best prove successful but ineffective in terms of cost and inconvenience to the patient.

In this chapter specific aspects of the history and physical examination, as they relate to myopathic disorders, will be discussed. These comments are intended to supplement a basic knowledge of clinical skills and not to provide an all-encompassing review of methods of clinical evaluation. The aim is to provide practical advice that will be of benefit at the bedside. Aspects of differential diagnosis will be discussed throughout the chapter and summarised at the end, and these later comments will lead into the following chapter which is concerned with investigative methods.

Clinical history

By convention, symptoms are what the patient complains of and signs are what the examiner observes and demonstrates. Some symptoms are not amenable to direct observation or quantitation; for example pain and some forms of fatigue. Some abnormal physical signs do not give rise to symptoms; for example some forms of myotonia and other disorders of muscle fibre relaxation. Conversely, many symptoms are also signs; notably wasting, weakness and various forms of involuntary muscle activity. The discussion of those features that can be both symptoms and signs will therefore be split between this section on the clinical history and the following on physical examination.

Skeletal muscle has only a limited repertoire of responses to a wide range of diseases and insults. The patient may complain of pain in the muscle, either at rest or on exercise, notice muscle enlargement or thinning, see and feel involuntary movements, be aware of weakness, or experience fatigue. Such muscle-related symptoms will be discussed first. Symptoms relating to organ systems other than skeletal muscle will be considered next. Such symptoms may point to a multisystem disorder of which myopathy is just a part, or a primary myopathic disorder may rarely have secondary effects elsewhere (e.g. renal failure due to myoglobinuria). The patient's past medical history, their family history, and their history of exposure to drugs and toxins may all provide vital clues that will help towards a diagnosis. In general, the history will provide more clues to the diagnosis than will the physical examination.

Table 1.1 *Myopathies that can often be diagnosed, or at least strongly suspected, at the bedside*

- Duchenne muscular dystrophy
- Emery-Dreifuss syndrome
- Facioscapulohumeral muscular dystrophy
- Oculopharyngeal muscular dystrophy
- Rigid spine syndrome
- Myotonic dystrophy
- Myotonia congenita
- Dermatomyositis
- Inclusion body myositis
- Some endocrine myopathies
- Some mitochondrial cytopathies
- Acid maltase deficiency (if there is diaphragmatic involvement)

Muscle-related symptoms

Pain

It is helpful to distinguish between causes of localised and generalised pain (Tables 1.2 & 1.3), and between pain that is present at rest (most of the conditions listed in Tables 1.2 & 1.3) and that which comes on during exercise (Table 1.4). Note that these are not all primary myopathic disorders, but all are conditions in which the patient perceives the pain as being in muscle. Numerous drugs may cause an acute or subacute painful myopathy (Table 1.5). The pathophysiological mechanisms associated with muscle pain are poorly understood. Chemical mediators as well as mechanical factors are involved. The nerve fibres conveying pain sensation are thinly myelinated or unmyelinated.

Table 1.2 *Disorders causing localized muscle pain (but not necessarily primary myopathic disorders)*
• Trauma (including compartment syndromes)
• Ischaemia
• Infection
– bacterial
– parasitic
• Metabolic and toxic myopathies
– acute alcoholic myopathy
– some glycogenoses
• Inflammation
– sarcoidosis
– eosinophilic fasciitis
• Neuralgic amyotrophy
• Focal (compressive and ischaemic) peripheral nerve lesions

Table 1.3 *Disorders causing generalised muscle pain (but not necessarily primary myopathic disorders)*
• Dermatomyositis & polymyositis (if acute/subacute)
• Infections
– viral (e.g. coxsackie, poliomyelitis)
– toxoplasmosis
• Drug-induced myopathies (see Table 1.5)
• Steroid withdrawal
• Metabolic myopathies
– metabolic bone disease
– hypothyroid myopathy
– carnitine palmitoyltransferase deficiency (CPT) deficiency
– acute alcoholic myopathy
• Polymyalgia rheumatica
• Eosinophilia-myalgia syndrome
• Connective tissue disorders
• Guillain-Barré syndrome
• Porphyria
• Amyotrophic lateral sclerosis
• Parkinson's disease
• In association with fever

Table 1.4 *Disorders associated with exercise-induced muscle pain*
• Ischaemia (claudication)
• Muscular dystrophies
– Duchenne
– Becker
• Metabolic myopathies
– glycogenoses
– mitochondrial cytopathies
– carnitine palmitoyltransferase deficiency (CPT) deficiency
– Brody's syndrome
• Tubular aggregate myopathy
• Dermatomyositis

Table 1.5 *Commonly used drugs that cause painful myopathy*

Amiodarone	Ciclosporin	Gemfibrozil
Labetalol	D-penicillamine	L-tryptophan
Cimetidine	EACA	Gold
Lovastatin	Procainamide	Vincristine
Clofibrate	Emetine	Heroin
Nifedipine	Salbutamol	Zidovudine

Muscle pain (myalgia) is an extremely common symptom in muscle clinics. It is often a major feature of the chronic fatigue syndrome, in which in the majority of patients there is no evidence of muscle pathology. If pain is the sole complaint and the history and physical examination fail to reveal a cause, then further investigation is often unrewarding.

Cramps, contractures, delayed relaxation and myotonia

Cramps

Common-or-garden muscle cramps are neurogenic in origin and thus not generally associated with primary muscle disorders. Motor nerve hyperactivity causes painful muscle contraction and neurophysiological studies in an attack show motor unit discharges at a frequency of several hundred Hertz. Predisposing factors include systemic metabolic disturbances and hypothyroidism. Considering potential differential diagnoses, it should be noted that anterior horn cell disorders, radiculopathies, and peripheral neuropathies may all be associated with cramps.

Two other disorders in which there is muscle over-activity secondary to neurogenic hyperactivity are neuromyotonia and stiff-man syndrome. Neuro-myotonia is characterised by stiffness, cramps and myokymia. Some patients have increased sweating and some have sensory symptoms. It may be associated with a variety of inherited and acquired disorders and there is strong evidence that autoimmunity is involved in at least some acquired cases. In stiff-man syndrome it is mainly the axial muscles that are involved. Spasms and stiffness give rise to spinal deformity and an abnormal gait. EMG shows continuous motor unit activity in affected muscles. Again, there is strong evidence for an autoimmune basis, with involvement of GABAergic pathways.

Contracture

The term "muscle contracture" is used in two quite different senses. In many chronic neurogenic and myopathic disorders there is shortening of muscles and an inability to passively stretch the muscle to its proper length (sometimes referred to as fixed contracture). This is caused by progressive fibrosis of the muscle and contributing factors include the disease process within the muscle itself and weakness of the antagonistic muscle. Such fixed contractures are usually a late feature of the disease, but there are some muscle disorders in which contractures are an early and often striking feature, and in which both the limbs and spine may be affected. These include Emery-Dreifuss muscular dystrophy (Figure 1.1), Bethlem myopathy, and the rigid-spine syndrome. Such contractures are of course electrically silent. It is important to distinguish muscle contracture from joint ankylosis.

The term contracture is also used to describe electrically silent active muscle contraction. This is seen characteristically in metabolic myopathies associated with disturbed glycogen or glucose metabolism, and in the even rarer disorders Brody's syndrome and the rippling muscle syndrome. In the muscle glycogenoses the contractures are painful, associated with muscle fibre damage and the risk of myoglobinuria, and are

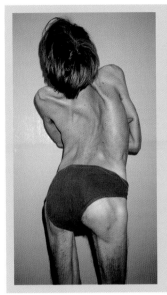

Figure 1.1
Autosomal dominant Emery-Dreifuss syndrome, demonstrating spinal contractures.

presumed to relate to a critical disturbance of high-energy metabolic pathways, although this has not been proven.

In Brody's syndrome, which is an extremely rare disorder caused by a deficiency of sarcoplasmic reticulum calcium-ATPase, there is exercise-induced stiffness and cramping, and slowness of muscle relaxation. Rippling muscle syndrome is a rare sporadic or dominantly inherited disorder in which patients complain of stiffness, and on examination stretching or percussion of muscle sets off ripples.

Myotonia

Myotonia is caused by recurrent depolarisation of the muscle fibre membrane and is characterised electrically by waxing and waning rhythmical discharges. The clinical correlates are muscle stiffness and slowness of relaxation, evident after voluntary contraction or percussion of the muscle. Myotonia is seen in three main clinical settings. In myotonic dystrophy the patient may complain of difficulty releasing objects after a firm grasp (Figure 1.2) or, less specifically, of stiffness of their hands and forearms. The myotonia may also affect tongue movements and chewing. In general, in myotonic dystrophy, weakness is more of a problem than myotonia and the myotonia may be asymptomatic even if very evident on examination. In myotonia congenita (chloride channelopathy) there is severe generalised myotonia. It is worse after rest, and on standing from sitting or when starting to walk the stiffness in the leg muscles may cause the patient to

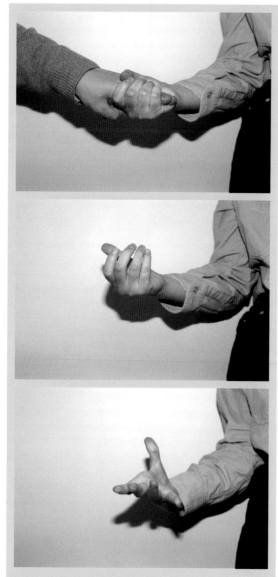

Figure 1.2 Grip myotonia in myotonic dystrophy. The patient was asked to grip the examiner's fingers tightly for 5 s, and then to release as rapidly as possible - subsequent pictures taken at 3 s intervals.

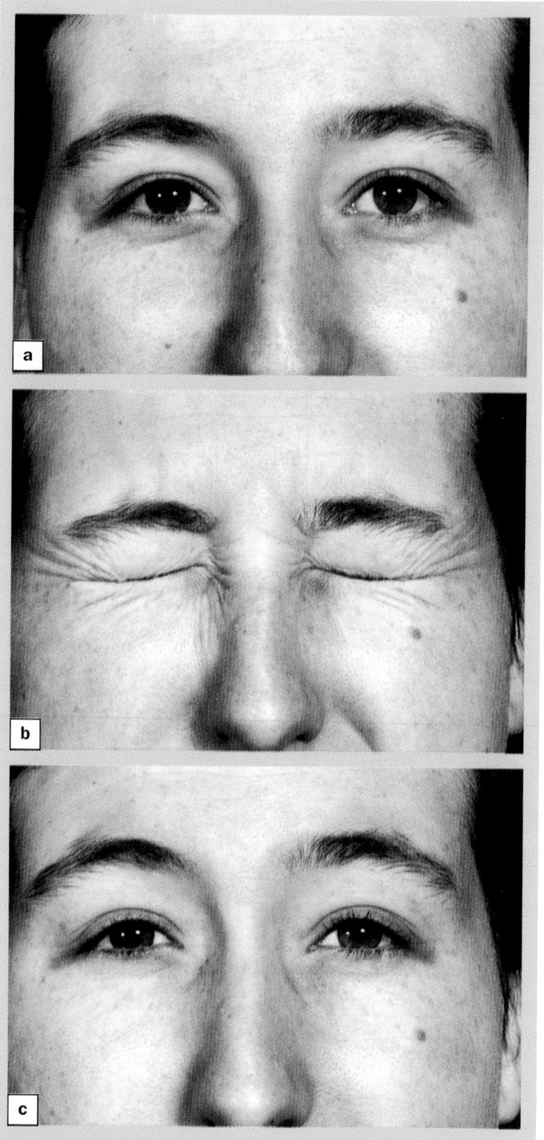

Figure 1.3 Myotonia congenita. The patient was asked to close her eyes tightly (b) for 3 s, and then to open them wide as rapidly as possible – the delayed relaxation (3(c), picture taken 3 s after command to open eyes) is apparent.

fall. There may be marked grip myotonia. A severe episode of myotonia may be followed by transient weakness of the affected muscle. The facial muscles are involved and an appearance like blepharospasm may be seen after forceful eye-closure (Figure 1.3). In the sodium channelopathies (paramyotonia congenita and hyperkalaemic periodic paralysis) the myotonia may be exacerbated by continuing activity (paradoxical myoto-

nia) whereas in the other forms described above it tends to ease. It may also be markedly exacerbated by cold. The facial, forearm and hand muscles tend to be the most affected.

Wasting and enlargement

Muscle wasting is not a very common presenting symptom of primary myopathic disorders although it may become very evident to the patient as the disease progresses. Early wasting is difficult for the patient and the examiner to see if the subcutaneous adipose tissue is plentiful (women and the obese). In the early stages of some diseases, particularly dystrophies, the wasting may be very focal within individual muscles. Sometimes there can be a bizarre appearance with focal atrophy and hypertrophy within one muscle. At a first approximation the degree of wasting parallels the degree of weakness in neurogenic disorders whereas in myopathies, particularly in the earlier stages, wasting may be slight or absent even in the presence of severe weakness. There are many exceptions to this generalisation and to the summary given in Table 1.6.

Muscle hypertrophy, either focal or generalised, is seen in a number of neuromuscular disorders (Table 1.7). True hypertrophy, a form of work hypertrophy of the muscle fibres secondary to repetitive activity, is seen in some cases of myotonia congenita (Figure 1.4) and neuromyotonia. This may be relevant in some of the other conditions listed in Table 1.7 but more frequently the enlargement is better termed pseudo-hypertrophy and is due to replacement of damaged muscle fibres by fat and connective tissue.

Weakness

This is by far the commonest presenting symptom of muscle disease. Patients may use the term rather loosely and as the history unfolds it often turns out

---

Table 1.6 Neuromuscular disorders and the associated degree of muscle wasting

Little wasting

Myasthenia gravis

Dermatomyositis/polymyositis

Many metabolic myopathies

Channelopathies

Upper motor neurone disorders

Wasting

Anterior horn cell disorders - amyotrophic lateral sclerosis (ALS), spinal muscular atrophy (SMA), poliomyelitis

Peripheral neuropathies

Congenital myopathies

Muscular dystrophies

Myotonic dystrophy

Distal myopathies

Table 1.7 Neuromuscular disorders associated with muscle hypertrophy or pseudohypertrophy

Muscular dystrophies

   – Duchenne/Becker

   – Manifesting carriers of Duchenne

   – Limb-girdle dystrophies

Myotonia congenita

Neuromyotonia

Spinal muscular atrophy

Spinal nerve root compression (e.g. S1 root and calf hypertrophy)

Debrancher enzyme deficiency

Cysticercosis

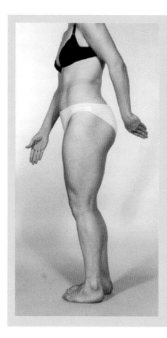

Figure 1.4 Myotonia congenita - note the generalised muscle hypertrophy.

---

that the patient is not describing weakness, as the physician understands it, but rather is complaining of non-specific fatigue, restriction of movement due to some mechanical problem or even sensory disturbance. Conversely, they may use words such as deadness, heaviness or even numbness to describe what is simply weakness. It is important to try to date the onset of weakness but this may be difficult, particularly in very slowly progressive disorders that have their onset in childhood (see below). The weakness may be static, as in some congenital neuromuscular disorders, or progressive, in which case an estimate of the rate of progression must be made. It may be fluctuating, as in myasthenic disorders, intermittent as in periodic paralysis and some myotonic disorders, or exercise-related as in many metabolic disorders. Specific symptoms relating to weakness in particular areas are discussed below.

Weakness of cranial nerve innervated muscles
Patients may complain of ptosis because of the cosmetic appearance or because it is severe enough to cover the pupil and obscure vision. Weakness of the extra-ocular muscles may cause diplopia. Variable ptosis and diplopia are characteristic of myasthenia gravis. Constant ptosis is seen in myotonic dystrophy, mitochondrial cytopathies, oculopharyngeal muscular dystrophy and a number of congenital neuromuscular syndromes. In mitochondrial disorders, despite severe restriction of eye-movements, diplopia is uncommon. Diplopia is rare in oculopharyngeal muscular dystrophy and in myotonic dystrophy. In thyroid ophthalmopathy ptosis and diplopia may be constant or fluctuating.

Facial weakness in myopathic disorders is usually bilateral and symmetrical. Because of the symmetry it is less evident to the patient and to lay or medical observers than unilateral facial weakness. Frequently, patients are asymptomatic even when examination shows very evident weakness. Specific enquiry may elicit a history of difficulty blowing up balloons or drinking through a straw. One of our patients, with facioscapulohumeral muscular dystrophy, was first aware of facial weakness when he was unable to seal his lips around a police breathalyser device - to the disbelief of the observers. Severe facial weakness contributes towards dysarthria, although in such situations there is often associated weakness of other bulbar muscles.

Weakness of limb muscles
Aspects of the history will point to whether the weakness is predominantly proximal or distal. Proximal upper limb weakness causes difficulties with activities performed above shoulder height, such as reaching up to shelves, hanging out washing and hair grooming. Distal upper limb weakness leads to complaints relating to grip and is seen most strikingly in those disorders that have distal weakness as an early feature, such as myotonic dystrophy, inclusion body myositis and the relatively rare distal myopathies. In the lower limbs proximal weakness in the early stages causes problems climbing stairs and getting up from chairs (particularly low ones) and later, when more severe, leads to gait disturbance. Selective weakness of quadriceps is seen in a number of disorders, most notably inclusion body myositis, and patients will often complain of falls due to their "knees giving way". Distal lower limb weakness causes foot-drop and the patient complains of "catching" their toes on minor irregularities of the ground surface, which may lead to falls. The combination of proximal and distal lower limb weakness, seen frequently in myotonic dystrophy and inclusion body myositis, leads to a history of tripping and falling due to foot-drop and then inability to get up without help due to the proximal weakness.

Respiratory muscles
Mild respiratory muscle weakness is asymptomatic and formal assessment (e.g. vital capacity) should be performed in all patients with diseases known to affect respiratory function in later stages. With increasing severity the patient complains of breathlessness on exertion and orthopnoea. The earliest symptoms of respiratory failure include nightmares, early morning headache and excessive daytime sleepiness. Acid maltase deficiency presents with respiratory failure in up to one-third of cases. Respiratory failure may also be seen during an episode of acute weakness in carnitine palmitoyltransferase deficiency. Respiratory failure, complicated by chest infection, is the commonest cause of death in Duchenne muscular dystrophy and is a frequent feature in later stages of rigid spine syndrome.

Myoglobinuria
Myoglobin is a haem protein that functions as a storage reservoir of oxygen and a carrier of oxygen from the cell membrane to mitochondria. Muscle membrane disruption allows release of myoglobin into the bloodstream (myoglobinaemia) and excretion into the urine (myoglobinuria). If released in significant quantities the myoglobin may cause renal failure from acute tubular necrosis. Treatment is supportive and forced alkaline diuresis is advocated but of unproven efficacy. Myoglobinuria is paralleled by an increase in the serum creatine kinase level. The patient notices myoglobinuria as discoloration of the urine which ranges from light brown to dark-brown/black. Such discoloration must be distinguished from other causes of pigmenturia, including drugs, haemolysis and porphyria.

Some of the more frequently encountered causes of myoglobinuria are listed in Table 1.8. More detailed reviews are available.

Table 1.8 *Causes of myoglobinuria*

Intensive exercise in normal individuals

Inherited myopathies

- Metabolic: glycogenoses (e.g. myophosphorylase deficiency); lipid disorders (e.g. carnitine palmitoyltransferase deficiency); malignant hyperthermia
- Dystrophic: Duchenne and Becker

Acquired myopathies

- Dermatomyositis and polymyositis
- Infections: viral; bacterial

Ischaemia and trauma

- Crush injury
- Status epilepticus
- Electric shock
- Arterial insufficiency

Drugs and toxins

- Alcohol
- Opiates
- Clofibrate
- Snake venom
- Bacterial toxins
- Carbon monoxide

Others

- Neuroleptic malignant syndrome
- Severe metabolic disturbances
- Fever and heat stroke
- Idiopathic

Table 1.9 *Myopathies associated with cardiac involvement*

Cardiomyopathy

- Duchenne and Becker muscular dystrophy
- Limb-girdle muscular dystrophy (rarely)
- Emery-Dreifuss syndrome (late)
- Dermatomyositis
- Infantile acid maltase deficiency
- Disorders of lipid metabolism
- Debranching enzyme deficiency
- Mitochondrial cytopathies
- Alcoholic cardiomyopathy
- Endocrine myopathies

Arrhythmias

- Myotonic dystrophy
- Emery-Dreifuss muscular dystrophy
- Mitochondrial cytopathies (particularly Kearns-Sayre syndrome)
- Periodic paralysis (particularly Andersen's syndrome)

tion death ensues from hepatic failure. Neonatal and childhood liver involvement, including recurrent Reye-like episodes, is common in disorders of carnitine metabolism and β-oxidation and may be seen with disorders of the mitochondrial respiratory chain.

Central nervous system

Mitochondrial respiratory chain disorders are frequently associated with central nervous system (CNS) involvement. CNS symptoms, including eye problems, may be the presenting feature and may

Table 1.10 *CNS and eye symptoms and signs in respiratory chain disorders*

- Stroke-like episodes
- Deafness
- Epilepsy
- Headache
- Ataxia
- Movement disorders
- Myoclonus
- Encephalopathy
- Dementia
- Dysphagia
- Pigmentary retinopathy
- Optic atrophy
- Progressive external ophthalmoplegia

Systemic symptoms
Heart

Cardiac involvement in myopathic disorders is common and may be the cause of significant morbidity and death. It is important to identify it early because some forms, particularly rhythm disorders, are amenable to therapy. Some disorders are particularly associated with myocardial disease (cardiomyopathy) whereas others more frequently cause arrhythmias (Table 1.9). The symptoms are those of cardiac failure and rhythm disturbance, respectively. Another important consideration is the development of cor pulmonale secondary to respiratory insufficiency.

Liver

Recurrent hypoglycaemia is a major feature of childhood, but not adult, onset debranching deficiency. In both, hepatomegaly may be noted as abdominal protuberance. In branching enzyme deficiency hepatomegaly is associated with ascites and without liver transplanta-

occur alone, without clinical evidence of muscle disease. Commonly seen symptoms and signs are summarised in Table 1.10.

Taken as a group, patients with Duchenne and Becker muscular dystrophy have on average a lower IQ than the normal population but this is not readily evident in the clinic. In myotonic dystrophy the lower IQ of the patient population is much more apparent, although many patients are of normal intellect. All patients with congenital myotonic dystrophy have a reduced IQ and often have quite severe learning difficulties. A lower than average IQ is also a feature of a number of congenital myopathies.

Peripheral nervous system

Disorders that are confined to skeletal muscle would not be expected to cause sensory symptoms but patients often use words that the unwary clinician might take to indicate peripheral nerve involvement. Thus, what is in fact just weakness may be described as deadness or numbness. They may even say that touching the affected part does not produce a normal sensation. Conversely, there are many disorders that involve muscle and nerve, leading to symptoms relating to both (Table 1.11), so that a history of sensory dysfunction must be sought.

Eyes

Ptosis and disorders of eye movements have been discussed above. Pigmentary retinopathy and optic

Table 1.11 Disorders that can affect both skeletal muscle and peripheral nerves

- Alcohol
- Amyloidosis
- Chronic renal failure
- Collagen vascular disorders
    - Rheumatoid arthritis
    - Systemic lupus erythematosus
- Drugs
    - Gold
    - Vincristine
- Endocrinopathies
    - Acromegaly
    - Hypothyroidism
- Malnutrition
- Paraneoplastic syndromes
- Sarcoidosis
- Vasculitides

Table 1.12 Endocrine disorders that can cause a myopathy

- Hypothyroidism
- Hyperthyroidism
- Graves' ophthalmopathy
- Cushing's syndrome
- Addison's disease
- Hyperparathyroidism
- Hypoparathyroidism
- Acromegaly
- Hypopituitarism
- Primary hyperaldosteronism
- Phaeochromocytoma

atrophy are commonly seen in patients with mitochondrial disorders but symptomatic impairment of vision is relatively unusual. Eye involvement, sometimes with severe visual failure, may be seen in some congenital muscular dystrophies.

Endocrine

Many (indeed most) endocrine disorders may cause a myopathy (Table 1.12), usually proximal and affecting the pelvic more than the shoulder girdle. The history must therefore seek symptoms of any such primary underlying endocrine disorder. Myasthenia gravis is associated with an increased incidence of thyroid dysfunction, the onset of which may exacerbate the myasthenia. Mitochondrial cytopathies have been linked with several endocrine disorders, including diabetes mellitus. A specific form of periodic paralysis is linked to hyperthyroidism.

Kidney

Myoglobinuria as a cause of renal damage has already been discussed. Chronic renal failure from whatever cause, dialysis and renal tubular acidosis can cause myopathy through several mechanisms.

Gastrointestinal system

Many neuromuscular disorders can affect the alimentary tract and a number of bowel disorders can cause myopathy. Malabsorption from whatever cause may cause myopathy secondary to osteomalacia. Dysphagia is a common symptom of neuromuscular disease and may relate to weakness of the pharyngeal muscles and to oesophageal dysmotility. Cough and symptoms relating to aspiration may be secondary features. Gastric stasis, pseudo-obstruction of the bowel and constipation may be due to immobility caused by the generalised neuromuscular disorder, or to direct involvement of smooth muscle. In myotonic dystrophy, symptoms akin to irritable bowel syndrome, and faecal soiling in childhood, are common. In the rare MNGIE syndrome (mitochondrial myopathy, peripheral neuropathy, gastrointestinal disease and encephalopathy) nausea, vomiting and diarrhoea are due to gut dysmotility.

Blood

Haemolytic anaemia is a feature of several of the disorders of glycogen/glucose metabolism, most notably phosphofructokinase deficiency. Clinical accompaniments are unusual except for jaundice, which is seen in about one-quarter of cases.

Skin

Cutaneous involvement is seen in most, but not all, cases of dermatomyositis. Raynaud's phenomenon is also common in this disorder. Lipomatosis is a rare feature in mitochondrial disorders.

Past medical history

Information about the past medical history obviously comes from the patient, or in the case of a child from the parents, but may need to be supplemented, or the accuracy checked, by reference to the family doctor or other medical records.

Related disorders

This should be relatively straightforward; one is simply trying to identify any pre-existing disorder, whether active or otherwise, that may give a clue as to the cause of the present neuromuscular problem. However, patients may forget to mention even persisting medical problems (such as hypertension or diabetes) and so specific enquiry may need to be made. It may be the disorder itself that is of interest, or its treatment.

Anaesthetic history

Many neuromuscular disorders affect the respiratory muscles but this may be asymptomatic in the early stages of the disease. Anaesthesia may expose the weakness and so sometimes a history of the patient being "difficult to wake up", or needing a prolonged period of assisted ventilation, after anaesthesia for an unrelated complaint is identified. Such a history is heard most often from patients with myotonic dystrophy who at the time of surgery did not know that they had the condition and so could not warn the anaes-

thetist. Myasthenia gravis presents problems with respect to both anaesthetic agents and neuromuscular blocking drugs. Anaesthesia may also precipitate cardiac dysrhythmia and again patients with myotonic dystrophy are at particular risk.

Malignant hyperthermia may occur in apparent isolation or in association with known central core disease. Patients with Duchenne/Becker muscular dystrophy may also be at risk of anaesthesia-induced hyperthermic reactions.

Family history

Obtaining an accurate family history can involve a great deal of work. The patient may know that another family member had problems with mobility (e.g. needed walking aids or a wheelchair), or that the appearance of their musculature was abnormal, but not have accurate information about the diagnosis. In some families, and particularly in older generations, there appears to be reluctance to discuss such matters openly. Further information may have to be obtained from other family members and medical records, although both sources can be unreliable. Remember also that prior to the 1960s diagnostic methods were limited and distinction between myopathic and neurogenic disorders may not have been possible. Nonspecific diagnoses such as muscular atrophy abounded.

Two other situations require particular caution. Some autosomal dominant neuromuscular disorders (e.g. facioscapulohumeral muscular dystrophy) show considerable variability, even within a family, and an affected parent may be or have been asymptomatic, so that no family history is evident. Particularly dramatic examples of this phenomenon are seen in conditions which show genetic anticipation, of which the commonest is myotonic dystrophy. If an inherited disorder is being considered and the parents are still alive, they should be examined even if reported to be asymptomatic. This is particularly important if genetic counselling is an issue. The other potential catch arises with X-linked disorders such as Duchenne and Becker muscular dystrophy. Depending on the family structure there may be several generations containing no affected males. Furthermore it must be remembered that for these particular disorders the new-mutation rate is about 30%.

Drugs and toxins

Many drugs, both prescribed and available over-the-counter, are known to be capable of causing a myopathy. The commoner culprits causing painful and

Table 1.13 *Commonly used drugs that cause painless myopathy*

- Amiodarone
- Chloroquine
- Colchicine
- Corticosteroids
- Heroin
- Hypokalaemia-inducing drugs (e.g. diuretics)
- Perhexiline

Table 1.14 *Muscles/actions that should be assessed in all patients with suspected neuromuscular disease*

- Cranial nerve innervated muscles
  - Eyelid elevation
  - Eye movement
  - Facial muscles
  - Palatal movements
  - Neck flexion/extension
  - Shoulder shrugging
  - Tongue movements
- Limbs and trunk
  - Scapula fixation
  - Shoulder abduction & adduction
  - Elbow flexion and extension
  - Wrist flexion and extension
  - Finger flexion, extension & abduction
  - Hip flexion and extension
  - Knee flexion and extension
  - Ankle dorsiflexion and plantar flexion
  - Trunk sitting from lying
  - Gait: assess walking, running, walking on heels and tip-toe
- Respiratory muscles
  - Diaphragm movement on inspiration

painless myopathy are listed in Tables 1.5 and 1.13 respectively. Their consumption is likely to be identified fairly readily, but the usage of illicit drugs may require more tenacious questioning. The true level of alcohol consumption may also be difficult to assess.

Physical examination

Given the associations between myopathies and general medical disorders discussed above it is readily apparent that physical examination must encompass all organ systems and not be confined to assessment of the muscles alone. This section will focus on a few particular aspects of the examination, perhaps what could be called tricks of the trade, and will not attempt to cover basic techniques, which are detailed in many texts. There is inevitably overlap between this section and the earlier part of this chapter on the Clinical History.

Skeletal muscle

We will start with comments on examination of the skeletal muscles and then discuss assessment of the central and peripheral nervous systems, although in practice this is not the order at the bedside. These will be followed by brief comments on general examination.

Inspection

There is a widespread tendency to rush inspection. The patient should be adequately undressed and the limb under inspection should be relaxed. If the patient is having to make an effort to support a limb in an uncomfortable position voluntary twitches may be misinterpreted as fasciculation. The texture of muscles, wasting and hypertrophy, and involuntary movements (e.g. fasciculation, rippling, myokymia, neuromyotonia) are noted, as are skeletal deformities such as pes

cavus and kyphoscoliosis. At this stage one may also look for percussion phenomena, as described below.

Weakness

It is convenient to think in terms of the cranial nerve innervated muscles, the limb and trunk muscles and the respiratory muscles. The symptoms associated with weakness in each of these areas have been discussed above and they point towards the likely findings on physical examination. There are some muscles (or more specifically actions or movements) that should be assessed in every patient presenting with a suspected neuromuscular disorder (Table 1.14). Additional muscles will need to be tested, as indicated by the presenting symptomatology and the findings on this basic assessment. Thus, in proximal myopathies one would want to examine other peri-scapular and shoulder muscles, such as the spinati, and other muscles around the hips, such as those involved with abduction, adduction and rotation. Highly selective involvement of specific muscles in the same anatomical area is typical of many of the muscular dystrophies (e.g. in facioscapulohumeral dystrophy biceps and triceps are affected but deltoid is spared). Likewise, if there is evidence of distal weakness other distal muscles and movements should be examined, such as the long finger flexors and extensors, small hand muscles, ankle eversion and inversion and the intrinsic muscles of the feet.

Cranial nerve innervated muscle

Ptosis and external ophthalmoplegia have been discussed above. It is important to remember to look for fatigue of eyelid elevation and of eye-movements as well as absolute restriction of movement.

Mild symmetrical bilateral facial weakness is easily missed. The most sensitive test is to ask the patient to close their eyes tightly - failure to bury the eyelashes completely is indicative of weakness (Figure 1.5). This is a more sensitive test than trying to force open the eyelids with your thumbs, as well as being kinder to the patient.

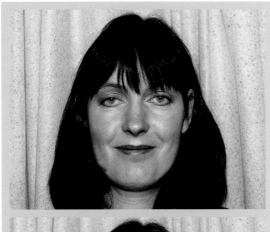
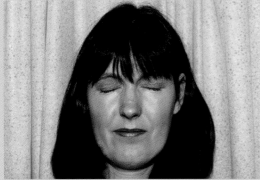

Figure 1.5 Bilateral facial weakness. The patient has central core disease. She is attempting to forcibly close her eyes, but is unable to fully bury her eyelashes.

In many neuromuscular disorders there is weakness of neck flexion, less frequently of neck extension. It is better to think of the movement of neck flexion rather than specifically of the action of the sternomastoid muscles, for several additional muscles are involved. This pattern of neck flexion weakness, sometimes marked, with normal extension is seen in many conditions but particularly myotonic dystrophy, myasthenia gravis and inflammatory myopathies. In some patients with myasthenia or myositis, particularly if the condition was long-standing before treatment became effective, weakness of neck flexion persists when all other evidence of weakness has resolved. Weakness of extension more than flexion is much less common but may be seen in myasthenia gravis, myositis, myotonic dystrophy, motor neurone disease and the illustratively labelled "dropped head syndrome".

Swallowing may be assessed subjectively by simply observing the patient eating and drinking. More objectively the time taken to swallow a certain volume of fluid, and the number of swallows taken, may be recorded.

Limb and trunk muscles

As is stated many times throughout this book, the pattern of muscle weakness may provide a strong clue to the diagnosis. Table 1.14 shows the muscles and movements that should be examined in every patient presenting with a neuromuscular problem and the findings on this basic screening, as well as the patients specific symptoms, will indicate if other muscles need to be tested.

We often want to record objectively the degree of weakness, either to enable us to plot the rate of deterioration in untreatable disorders and thus follow their natural history or, more importantly, to assess response to therapy in treatable conditions such as the inflammatory myopathies. Although much needed, simple reproducible tests have proved rather elusive. By far the most widely used, but amongst the least useful, is the Medical Research Council (MRC) scale (Table 1.15). Although the expansion of Grade 4 is of some value there is considerable inter- and intra-observer variability. Laboratory testing may be more reproducible but due to lack of availability is of little use in everyday practice.

However, there are a number of simple bedside tests which, even if not truly quantitative, give a clear picture of whether the weakness is worsening or improving and which are not subject to observer variability (Table 1.16). Which of these tests are

Table 1.15 *MRC scale of muscle strength. (Reproduced from* Aids to the examination of the peripheral nervous system. *London: Baillière Tindall, 1986.)*

Grade 0	No contraction
Grade 1	Flicker of contraction
Grade 2	Active movement, with gravity eliminated
Grade 3	Active movement against gravity
Grade 4–	Active movement against slight resistance
Grade 4	Active movement against moderate resistance
Grade 4+	Active movement against strong resistance
Grade 5	Normal power

Table 1.16 *Simple, semi-quantitative, bedside tests of muscle function*

- Lying supine on couch – lifting head
- Lying supine on couch – lifting lower limb straight up. Measure heel-couch distance
- Sitting up from lying
- Standing up from "standard" chair ⎱ Without use of
- Rising from a squat ⎰ upper limbs
- Ability to run and hop
- Ability to walk on heels and on tip-toe
- Ability to climb steps in "child" or "adult" fashion (one at a time or one after another)
- Time to walk a specific distance

applicable depends upon the severity of the weakness. A patient with mild proximal lower limb weakness may be able to walk normally and to get up from a chair without having to push with the upper limbs, but may not be able to rise from a squat. If, six months later, the subject can rise from a squat then it is very good evidence that improvement has occurred, whereas if rising from a chair as well as rising from a squat now proves impossible then there has been deterioration. Somebody with more severe weakness might only be able to lift a heel 50cm off the couch while lying supine. If at a later date they cannot quite lift the heel from the sheet then clearly they are weaker.

Weakness of truncal muscles may be evident when the patient tries to sit up from lying. With greater weakness there may be spinal deformity in the form of scoliosis or kyphosis. An exaggerated lumbar lordosis is common in Duchenne/Becker and other forms of limb-girdle muscular dystrophy. Scoliosis is common

in a number of congenital myopathies and in hereditary motor and sensory neuropathy.

Fatigue, a pronounced feature in myasthenia gravis and some metabolic myopathies, may be assessed in a number of ways. Shoulder abduction may be shown to fatigue with sustained pressure from the examiner. After a few attempts it may become impossible for the patient to rise from a squat.

Respiratory muscles
Patient may have advanced respiratory muscle insufficiency before they develop overt symptoms of respiratory failure and before signs at the bedside become obvious. It is therefore imperative to assess respiratory function, particularly in those patients with a neuromuscular disorder known to be associated with respiratory muscle (usually the diaphragm) weakness. The most frequently encountered are Guillain-Barré syndrome, motor neurone disease, Duchenne and Becker muscular dystrophy, acid maltase deficiency, myotonic dystrophy and several of the congenital myopathies. Paradoxical movement of the abdominal wall is a relatively late feature. On inspiration the upper abdomen normally moves outwards on inspiration as the diaphragm descends. If the diaphragm is weak it is drawn up on inspiration, by the negative intrathoracic pressure, and the abdominal wall moves inwards. The best test of respiratory muscle function at the bedside is measurement of the forced vital capacity, not peak flow.

Reflexes
In general the tendon reflexes are preserved in myopathies although they may be lost when wasting and weakness are advanced. In neuropathies reflex loss tends to occur early. There are frequent exceptions to these generalisations. In myasthenia gravis the reflexes are often relatively brisk. In the Lambert-Eaton myasthenic syndrome an absent tendon reflex may appear after sustained contraction of the appropriate muscle - so-called potentiation of the reflex. In myxoedema one may see delayed relaxation of a reflex. This is perhaps most often described for the ankle jerk but is sometimes better seen with the supinator reflex.

Percussion phenomena and abnormal relaxation
By far the commonest of these is myotonia, usually associated with myotonic dystrophy. Myotonia congenita and sodium channelopathies are much less common, but in myotonia congenita the myotonia may be much more severe than in myotonic dystrophy. Grip myotonia is easily demonstrated by asking the

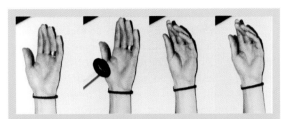

Figure 1.6 Percussion myotonia in a patient with myotonic dystrophy. A brisk tap with a tendon hammer of the thenar eminence causes muscle contraction followed by slow relaxation. Often it takes more than 5 s for full relaxation to occur.

patient to grip the examiner's fingers tightly for several seconds and then to release as rapidly as possible (Figure 1.2). Percussion myotonia is best seen by sharply tapping the thenar eminence with a tendon hammer (Figure 1.6). Myotonia is more widespread in myotonia congenita than in myotonic dystrophy, and may be demonstrated by percussing other muscles, such as quadriceps and deltoid. Exercise-induced stiffness and impaired relaxation, sometimes with cramps and myalgia, are a prominent feature in the very rare Brody's syndrome. Myoedema, or the mounding-phenomenon, is seen in myxoedema and severe malnutrition; after percussion of a muscle with a tendon hammer a ridge appears and may persist for many seconds.

Central nervous system (CNS)

A basic appraisal should of course be performed in all patients but a more detailed CNS examination is essential in patients suspected of having a metabolic myopathy, particularly a mitochondrial cytopathy (Table 1.10). Eye signs are common. The pigmentary retinopathy is mainly peripheral and it may be necessary to dilate the pupils to see it. Hearing loss may be mild and easily overlooked.

Peripheral nervous system

Examination of the peripheral nervous system is vital. Not only is the differential diagnosis likely to include neurogenic disorders but also a number of conditions can involve nerves as well as muscle (Table 1.11). Testing should include superficial sensation, joint-position and vibration sense. In some neurogenic disorders (e.g. Guillain-Barré syndrome) sensory symptoms and signs may be absent despite extensive motor involvement.

General examination

The need for a detailed general physical examination is self-evident from earlier comments. Cardiac involvement is common in neuromuscular disorders (Table 1.9). Apart from respiratory failure due to muscle weakness the lungs themselves may be involved (e.g. interstitial fibrosis in dermatomyositis). Abdominal examination may reveal hepatomegaly. Cutaneous manifestations are seen in dermatomyositis and other connective tissue disorders associated with muscle involvement and, rarely, in mitochondrial disorders. The manifestations of endocrine disorders, apart from evidence of a myopathy, are of course legion. In brief, one is looking for evidence of any systemic disorder that may be associated with myopathy.

Specific features in childhood

Disorders having an onset in early infancy and childhood cause particular problems for the assessor. There is the obvious difficulty that the patient cannot present his or her own history. The "standard" adult neurological physical assessment is not appropriate or applicable, particularly to very young children. An excellent review of the approach to neuromuscular problems in childhood is Dubowitz's classic monograph, which includes a useful structured questionnaire. Areas covered include pregnancy, labour, milestones, features of the presenting neuromuscular problem, and the past and family history.

In some congenital myopathies the mother may notice reduced foetal movements during the pregnancy. Perinatal features may include hypotonia (the "floppy baby"), and feeding and breathing difficulties. Weakness may first be evident as delayed motor milestones. It is very important, but can also very difficult, to try to determine the age of onset and whether the weakness is static, improving or progressive. It may take many years of observation before one can comment with any certainty on the rate of change, and thus the prognosis. The family may be able to comment on a change in appearance of the muscle, whether atrophy or hypertrophy. Even in very young children it may be evident that exercise induces pain in the muscles.

Listening carefully to the parents' description of their child's problems and watching the child at play will often be more revealing than a rigid approach using a structured interview and formal examination technique.

Differential diagnosis

Aspects of differential diagnosis have been considered throughout this chapter and will be discussed repeatedly in subsequent chapters when dealing with specific disorders. Two particular areas need to be addressed. Firstly, there is the question of differentiating between myopathies (i.e. primary disorders of muscle), neurogenic disorders (i.e. disorders affecting anterior horn cells or peripheral nerves) and disorders affecting the neuromuscular junction (myasthenic syndromes). Secondly, we need to be able to differentiate between different myopathies. An everyday example of the type of problem that we face is the patient who presents with weakness in limb-girdle distribution. The differential diagnosis (excluding CNS disorders) includes:

- Myopathies
  - muscular dystrophy (many types)
  - inflammatory myopathy (many types)
  - primary metabolic myopathy (many types)
  - secondary metabolic or endocrine myopathy (many types)
- Anterior horn cell disorders
  - spinal muscular atrophy (various types)
  - classical motor neurone disease
  - Kennedy's syndrome
- Peripheral neuropathies
  - inflammatory demyelinating polyradiculoneuropathies
  - metabolic causes (many).

The history and physical examination should reduce this formidable list to more manageable numbers, but even then it is not uncommon after clinical assessment alone to still harbour uncertainty as to whether one is dealing with a neurogenic or myopathic disorder. Selected investigations (described in the next chapter) will generally lead on to the correct diagnosis, but it would be honest to admit at this stage that even after very extensive investigation the diagnosis may remain elusive. Every neuromuscular clinic has a collection of patients patiently, or otherwise, awaiting a diagnostic label.

The most obvious features favouring a disorder of peripheral nerve, rather than a myopathy, are the presence of sensory symptoms and signs. However, there are many potential catches. Not all neuropathies always cause demonstrable sensory involvement. Prime examples include the acute and chronic forms of acquired demyelinating polyradiculoneuropathy, which thus enter the differential diagnosis of limb-girdle syndromes, and Charcot-Marie-Tooth syndrome which may mimic distal myopathies. Some diseases can directly affect both nerves and muscles. In any myopathy causing severe disability/immobility sensory symptoms may be due to simple compressive neuropathies. On examination, muscle wasting and depression of tendon reflexes are seen earlier in neurogenic disorders. Similarly, in anterior horn cell disorders suggestive features include cramps, fasciculation and early muscle wasting. Myasthenia gravis is characterised by fatigability and early involvement of the ocular and bulbar musculature, but differentiation from mitochondrial cytopathy can be very difficult.

Many aspects of the history and physical examination will help to discriminate between different myopathies. It goes without saying that a family history of an inherited neuromuscular disorder provides a powerful clue towards diagnosis, but beware of coincidences! Identification of a disorder known to be associated with muscle involvement, such as Cushing's syndrome, is obviously helpful. Age of onset is often of powerful discriminant value. Duchenne dystrophy doesn't present at age 15 years. Primary periodic paralyses don't present in old age. Oculopharyngeal muscular dystrophy rarely presents in early adult life, but mitochondrial external ophthalmoplegia can present at any age. The rate of progression may also be informative. Many congenital disorders are non-progressive, or change only very slowly with time. Inflammatory myopathies, but not dystrophies, may have a very acute onset with severe weakness developing within a matter of days. Metabolic disorders and channelopathies may cause slowly progressive weakness, over many decades, but with superimposed acute exacerbations. The pattern of weakness may be highly informative. Dystrophies tend to "pick out" certain muscles whereas inflammatory myopathies are rather less selective. Cardiac muscle and conduction tissues are only involved in certain myopathies. The many non-myopathic features associated with mitochondrial cytopathies have been reviewed above.

By the end of the interview and examination a short-list of diagnoses should have been achieved. The following chapter describes the investigations needed to reduce that number even further.

Selected further reading

Textbooks of muscle disease

Dubowitz V. *Muscle Disorders in Childhood*, 2nd ed. London: Saunders, 1995.

Engel AG, Franzini-Armstrong C (eds). *Myology*, 2nd edn. New York: McGraw-Hill, 1994.

Karpati G, Hilton-Jones D, Griggs R (eds). *Disorders of Voluntary Muscle*, 7th edn. Cambridge: Cambridge University Press, 2001.

Lane RJM. *Handbook of Muscle Disease*. New York: Marcel Dekker, 1996.

Specific disorders

Argov Z, Ruff R. Toxic and iatrogenic myopathies. In: Karpati G, Hilton-Jones D, Griggs R (eds). *Disorders of Voluntary Muscle*, 7th edn. Cambridge: Cambridge University Press, 2001.

Harper PS (ed). *Myotonic Dystrophy*, 2nd ed, vol 21. London: WB Saunders, 1989.

Hilton-Jones D, Squier M, Taylor D, Matthews P (eds). *Metabolic Myopathies*. London: WB Saunders, 1995.

Mullie MA, Harding AE, Petty RKH, Ikeda H, Morgan-Hughes JA, Sanders MD. The retinal manifestations of mitochondrial myopathy. *Arch Ophthalmol* 1985; 103: 1825–1830.

Petty RKH, Harding AE, Morgan-Hughes JA. The clinical features of mitochondrial myopathy. *Brain* 1986; 109: 915–938.

chapter 2

Investigation of muscle disease

The previous chapter concluded with the expectation that detailed clinical evaluation should have enabled the assessor to narrow down the differential diagnosis to a relatively short list of possibilities, and then that selective application of the investigations described in this chapter will lead to a precise diagnosis. Such often proves to be the case and perhaps the commonest course of events in general neuromuscular practice is: clinical assessment (which suggests a peripheral neuromuscular problem) → neurophysiology (which suggests a myopathy) → serum creatine kinase estimation (elevated) → muscle biopsy → DIAGNOSIS.

It is of course the exceptions and the rarer diagnoses that provide particular interest and sometimes a greater diagnostic challenge. Throughout this book the results of investigations will be discussed when considering individual disorders, but looking up information that way rather implies that the diagnosis has already been made! Much of this chapter is devoted to a review of the investigative techniques available, but it will start with an overview of possible approaches to particular clinical problems.

Approaches to investigation

Although this book is devoted to myopathies it has to be admitted that even after the most thorough clinical assessment it may not be possible, at the bed-side, to decide whether the patient has a myopathy or a neuropathy (or even a myasthenic syndrome), as was discussed in Chapter 1 when considering differential diagnosis. Presented with such uncertainty the most valuable initial investigations are likely to be estimation of the serum creatine kinase and neurophysiological studies. If these suggest a myopathic disorder, and there is no clinical or other information to suggest that the myopathy is secondary to a systemic disorder (such as an endocrinopathy), then it is probable that the disorder falls into one of the broad categories of primary myopathy listed in Table 2.1. Although

Table 2.1 *Major categories of primary muscle disease*

- Muscular dystrophies
- Congenital myopathy
- Myotonic dystrophy
- Inflammatory myopathies
- Primary metabolic myopathies
- Channelopathies

individual disorders within each category may have very specific test findings it is possible to make some useful generalisations as to the investigations that are most likely to be helpful in pursuing the diagnosis.

Before discussing these it is important to remember that tests may serve a number of different purposes. Some tests provide a specific diagnosis, obvious examples being enzyme assays in various metabolic disorders and DNA analysis in many genetic disorders. Others point towards the nature of the problem but not necessarily the exact diagnosis; e.g. an abnormal forearm exercise test or magnetic resonance spectroscopy study might indicate a glycogenolytic disorder but not the specific enzyme deficiency. Some tests, discussed later under the heading 'Ancillary investigations', may show important abnormalities that are a consequence of the primary disorder and which may influence management, but which in themselves do not provide a diagnosis; e.g. electrocardiography and echocardiography. Finally, there are investigations which, at least at present, can only be considered to be of research value; e.g. analysis of protein sub-units in mitochondrial disorders.

Tables 2.2-2.8 list investigations which are most likely to be of value in assessing particular diagnostic possibilities. These include those tests that may achieve a specific diagnosis as well as those which are less specific but which may more closely delineate the nature of the problem (e.g. forearm exercise test). Not included in the tables, but always performed in practice, is serum creatine kinase (CK) assay. It is an

Table 2.2 *Muscular dystrophies – major investigations*

- Muscle biopsy
  - Histology
  - Immunocytochemistry
  - Immunoblotting
- DNA studies

Table 2.3 *Myotonic dystrophy – major investigation*

- Gene analysis

Table 2.4 *Inflammatory myopathies – major investigations*

- Muscle biopsy
  - Histology
  - Immunocytochemistry
  - Electron microscopy
- Skin biopsy

Table 2.5 *Myopathies due to disorders of carbohydrate metabolism – major investigations*

- Forearm exercise test (assay lactate and ammonia)
- Magnetic resonance spectroscopy
- Muscle biopsy
  - Histochemistry
- Enzyme assay
  - Muscle
  - Blood cells
  - Fibroblasts
- Leucocyte glycogen storage
- DNA studies

Table 2.6 *Myopathies due to disorders of lipid metabolism – major investigations*

- Urinalysis
  - Organic acids
  - Acylcarnitines
- Tandem mass spectrometry
- Prolonged fasting (assay free fatty acids, lactate, pyruvate, uric acid, ammonia, ketone bodies, glucose, creatine kinase)
- Aerobic exercise (assay as above)
- Carnitine assay
  - Blood
- Muscle
- Enzyme assay
  - Muscle
  - Fibroblasts
  - Liver
- DNA studies

Table 2.7 *Mitochondrial cytopathies – major investigations*

- Resting blood lactate and pyruvate
- Aerobic exercise (assay lactate, pyruvate, ammonia, glucose)
- Muscle biopsy
  - Histochemistry
- Mitochondrial DNA studies
- Magnetic resonance spectroscopy

Table 2.8 *Channelopathies – major investigations*

- Neurophysiological studies
- Serum potassium changes during attacks (for periodic paralysis)
- Provocation tests (for periodic paralysis)
- Exercise testing
- DNA studies

often quoted generalisation that the CK is raised in myopathic disorders and normal in neuropathies, but there are many exceptions to this rule, as well as there being a number of disorders which are not primarily neuromuscular in which the CK is elevated. These issues are discussed later. Similarly, neurophysiological studies are not listed in most of the tables although frequently performed. While very useful for helping to distinguish between neurogenic and myopathic disorders, and for studying the channelopathies, they are of less value in the diagnosis of primary myopathies because other tests are more specific. Ancillary investigations, looking for abnormalities associated with the primary disorder but which in themselves are not specific, are discussed separately below.

Muscular dystrophies

In some of the muscular dystrophies (Table 2.2) the diagnosis may be made on the basis of clinical features and family history, without resorting to laboratory investigation (e.g. facioscapulohumeral and oculopharyngeal muscular dystrophy). Gene studies are becoming increasingly important and in some situations might arguably replace muscle biopsy (e.g. in a boy with characteristic features of Duchenne muscular dystrophy and a very high CK level). Routine histological and electron microscopy studies are rarely diagnostic, an exception being the characteristic 8.5 nm intranuclear filamentous inclusions seen in oculopharyngeal muscular dystrophy, although diagnosis is now based on DNA analysis. Immunocytochemistry and immunoblotting are major tools in the study of the dystrophinopathies (Duchenne and Becker), the limb-girdle dystrophies caused by deficiency of dystrophin-associated proteins, and some congenital dystrophies.

Myotonic dystrophy

Table 2.3 is included to emphasise that if myotonic dystrophy is suspected the appropriate, and definitive, investigation is gene analysis. Prior to the identification of the gene the most useful screening tests were electromyography and slit-lamp examination of the lenses (but not muscle biopsy) but these have now been superseded.

Inflammatory myopathies

In the idiopathic inflammatory myopathies (Table 2.4) the definitive investigation is muscle biopsy. Electromyography may be suggestive but is not diagnostic and, particularly in slowly progressive cases, serum CK may be normal. However, it must be remembered that inflammatory changes within muscle may be patchy and sampling-error can lead to a non-informative biopsy. Routine histology may be diagnostic but immunocytochemistry and electron microscopy (in inclusion body myositis) provide much useful additional information.

Metabolic myopathies

Metabolic myopathies (Tables 2.5-2.7) are rare and their investigation can be complex. Exercise tests, which are often badly performed and incorrectly interpreted, may be very useful in determining the site of metabolic dysfunction and as a prelude to more detailed biochemical investigation. Histochemical methods may sometimes demonstrate directly the enzyme deficiency or show accumulated products (e.g. glycogen, lipid) resulting from the blocked metabolic pathway. Enzyme assay may be performed on a sample from the biopsy. For those disorders in which the genetic defect is known, DNA analysis can usually be performed on a blood sample but at a research level RNA studies on muscle may be useful. An important exception is mitochondrial DNA deletion/duplication syndromes in which the genetic defect can only readily be detected in muscle, not lymphocytes.

Channelopathies

With respect to the channelopathies (Table 2.8) electromyography is useful, particularly in myotonic disorders. In the periodic paralyses monitoring serum potassium levels in attacks may be diagnostic and provocative tests can be very helpful, although somewhat hazardous. Direct gene analysis is rapidly becoming the investigation of choice.

Neurophysiology

Although many techniques are now available in clinical neurophysiology departments, those of everyday interest when considering neuromuscular disorders are nerve conduction studies (NCS), electromyography (EMG), and methods for studying neuromuscular transmission. The clinical overlap between anterior horn cell, motor neurone and peripheral nerve diseases (what are often called for simplicity neurogenic disorders), primary diseases of muscle (myopathic disorders), and myasthenic syndromes, has already been noted. It is often the case that EMG and NCS will strongly indicate whether one is dealing with a neurogenic or myopathic disorder, but it would be a gross oversimplification to say that these techniques always allow such a distinction to be made. It cannot be over-emphasised that the results must not be viewed in isolation but must be interpreted in the light of the clinical findings and the results of other tests.

Muscle fibre disease does not affect nerve conduction and so NCS would be expected to be normal. However, they are an important part of the overall evaluation of a suspected neuromuscular disorder. Furthermore, there are some diseases which mainly produce a myopathy but which may also be associated with a subclinical neuropathy (e.g. mitochondrial disorders, myotonic dystrophy). In EMG a needle is inserted into a muscle and muscle fibre action potentials are recorded from the extracellular space. Important techniques in the study of disorders of the neuromuscular junction include repetitive stimulation studies and assessment of jitter.

Table 2.9 *Principal electromyographic findings in neuromuscular disorders*

	Neurogenic	Myopathy	Myositis	Dystrophy	Myotonia
Insertional activity*	↑	N	↑	N	Myotonic discharges
Spontaneous activity	Fibrillations +ve sharp waves	N	Fibrillations +ve sharp waves	Fibrillations +ve sharp waves**	–
Motor unit potentials	Large amplitude Long duration	Low amplitude Short duration	Low amplitude Short duration	Low amplitude Short duration	Myotonic discharges
Interference pattern	Reduced	Early, full	Early, full	Early, full	Full

Insertional activity is reduced in severely atrophic or fibrotic muscle, whatever the initial pathological process.
** If there is active necrosis.

Electromyography

The most valuable technique in routine practice is concentric needle electrode electromyography. The EMG examination can be divided into four stages: assessment of insertional activity, identification of spontaneous activity, analysis of motor unit potentials, and assessment of the interference pattern. The particular patterns seen in neuromuscular disorders are discussed below and summarised in Table 2.9 and Figure 2.1.

Insertional activity

Needle insertion or movement induces a burst of high-frequency potentials, lasting a few hundred milliseconds, probably as the result of fibre damage caused by the needle. It is difficult to quantify. Decreased insertional activity is seen in fibrotic or severely atrophied muscle and during attacks of periodic paralysis. Increased activity is typical of denervation but may also be seen in inflammatory myopathies, myotonic disorders, acid maltase deficiency and hypothyroidism.

Spontaneous activity

Fibrillation potentials are spontaneous discharges (lasting 1-5ms) arising from single muscle fibres and probably reflect functional denervation of the fibre by disease of the muscle membrane at the end-plate zone. Positive sharp waves show an initial positive spike followed by a slower negative potential. Their origin is unclear but they generally have the same significance as fibrillation potentials and often occur together. They are typical of denervation but are also seen in inflammatory myopathies, dystrophies and a variety of endocrine and metabolic myopathies.

Fasciculation potentials are produced by the spontaneous discharge of muscle fibres of an entire motor unit, whereas fibrillation potentials and positive sharp waves arise from single fibres. They are usually associated with anterior horn cell disorders, particularly motor neurone disease, but may be seen in thyrotoxic myopathy (in which myokymia may also be seen).

Complex repetitive discharges (also known as bizarre high-frequency discharges) are prolonged bursts caused by the near-synchronous repetitive firing of a group of muscle fibres - over the loudspeaker they sound like a machine gun. They are very non-specific, being seen in association with denervation (including spinal muscular atrophy and Charcot–Marie–Tooth syndrome) and many myopathic disorders (e.g. inflammatory myopathies, dystrophies, hypothyroidism and acid maltase deficiency).

Myotonic discharges consist of trains of discharges, waxing and waning in frequency and amplitude, and sound like a dive-bomber over the loudspeaker. They correlate with the clinical myotonia seen in the various myotonic disorders but may also be seen in the absence of clinically evident myotonia in chronic denervation, acid maltase deficiency and hypothyroidism.

Motor unit potentials

A motor unit potential (MUP) is the summation of a number of single-fibre potentials arising within the same motor unit. Four characteristics of the MUP are useful diagnostically: amplitude, duration, number of phases and the stability of the waveform.

The amplitude depends upon the number of fibres discharging close to the needle tip. It tends to be small in myopathic disorders, because of loss of functional

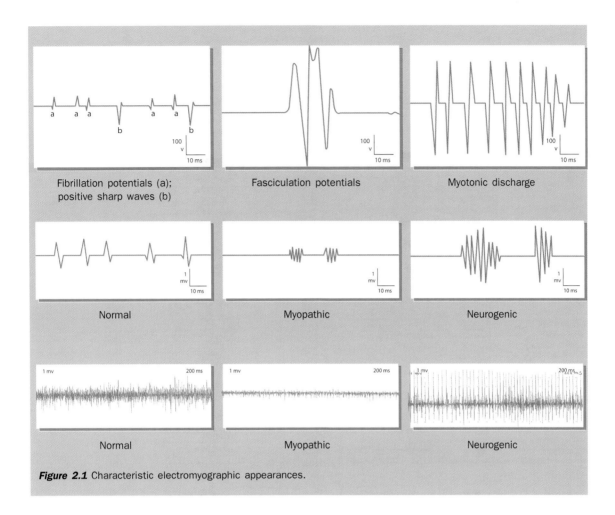

Figure 2.1 Characteristic electromyographic appearances.

fibres, and large in neurogenic disorders because collateral re-innervation produces an increased number of fibres within a motor unit. Because the size of the electrical field of an individual fibre is proportional to its diameter, large MUPs may be seen in myopathies associated with fibre hypertrophy (e.g. some dystrophies).

MUP duration reflects synchrony of firing of fibres within a motor unit and is determined by the length of terminal axon branches and the speed of propagation in these nerves and in the muscle fibres. The duration is prolonged in neurogenic disorders with re-innervation due to axonal sprouting, and reduced in myopathic disorders because of loss of functional muscle fibres.

MUPs are usually bi- or tri-phasic. A greater number of phases (polyphasic potentials) arises as a result of increased temporal dispersion of the firing of the fibres within a motor unit. This can be due to either altered innervation or to changes in the conductivity of muscle fibre membranes and thus polyphasia is seen in both neurogenic and myopathic disorders.

Normally, individual MUPs have a constant shape and amplitude. Slight variability from one moment to the next is called instability and this phenomenon has the same significance as increased jitter (discussed below). Instability is seen with disorders of the neuromuscular junction, in cases of rapid denervation, in the early stages of re-innervation, and in some inflammatory myopathies.

Interference pattern

With increasing effort of voluntary contraction the rate of firing of individual motor units increases and additional units become active (a process known as recruitment). The term interference pattern is used when it is no longer possible to identify individual MUPs in the summated response seen on the recording oscilloscope. In neurogenic disorders the remaining motor neurones have to fire faster than normal to achieve the required force. Even at maximum effort individual MUPs can still be identified and the interference pattern is said to be reduced. In myopathic disorders, the loss of fibres means that a greater number of units than normal needs to be active to generate a given force and so a more complex interference pattern develops at a lower force of contraction (early recruitment). Such early recruitment is also seen in neuromuscular junction transmission disorders.

Repetitive stimulation

Repetitive supra-maximal nerve stimulation and measurement of the evoked muscle action potential is a useful technique for studying neuromuscular junction transmission. In myasthenia gravis the characteristic response to 3 Hz stimulation is progressive reduction (decrement) in the amplitude of the compound muscle action potential (CMAP) from the first to the fourth or fifth stimulus, followed by partial recovery (Figure 2.2a). In the Lambert–Eaton myasthenic syndrome the resting CMAP amplitude is reduced and at slow rates of stimulation (e.g. 3 Hz) a decremental response is seen, as in myasthenia gravis. At higher rates (e.g. 20 Hz), or following brief voluntary contraction (post-tetanic potentiation), the CMAP amplitude shows a marked increase, in excess of 25% (Figure 2.2b).

Jitter

The single-fibre EMG electrode, as its name rather implies, was designed so that it would detect the local electrical fields of only a small number of muscle fibres (in contrast to the standard concentric electrode which responds to a large number of fibres). Such a needle can be positioned so that it detects the potentials from only two muscle fibres, each innervated by a terminal branch of the same axon. In response to nerve stimulation or voluntary contraction (as is more often used in clinical practice) these two fibres fire nearly, but not quite, simultaneously. The small time difference between the potentials is called the interpotential interval, and is in the order of a few tens of microseconds. This interval reflects the difference in conduction times along the two separate pathways of: terminal axon-neuromuscular junction-muscle fibre. Jitter is measured as the mean consecutive difference of successive interpotential intervals and is normally less than 50μs. The main source of jitter in normal muscles is neuromuscular transmission. It is increased in disorders of neuromuscular transmission. If the jitter value is very prolonged the phenomenon of blocking may be seen, when intermittently one of the two potentials fails to appear. Prolonged jitter may be seen in neuropathies with denervation and re-innerva-

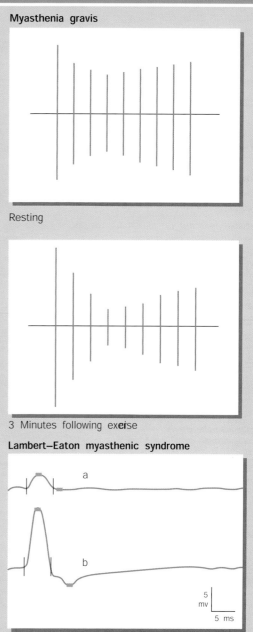

MYASTHENIA GRAVIS AND LAMBERT–EATON SYNDROME

Myasthenia gravis

Resting

3 Minutes following exeise

Lambert–Eaton myasthenic syndrome

a

b

5 mv

5 ms

Figure 2.2 Myasthenia gravis and Lambert–Eaton myasthenic syndrome. I) In myasthenia gravis, repetitive nerve stimulation at 3Hz produces a decremental response in the compound muscle action potential. II) In the Lambert–Eaton syndrome the compound muscle action potential at rest is small (a), but increases following 15 seconds maximal voluntary contraction (b).

tion, and in myopathies associated with damage to the neuromuscular region. Reduced jitter is seen in muscular dystrophies, arising from split muscle fibres, but this is of little clinical importance. Increased jitter occurs in mitochondrial cytopathies, which is important to remember when investigating patients with progressive external ophthalmoplegia in whom neuromuscular junction disorders enter the differential diagnosis.

Muscle imaging

There is no doubt that muscle imaging has its enthusiasts. Although in occasional patients it can prove invaluable it must be noted that the majority of patients, passing through a neuromuscular department do not require imaging and indeed many highly regarded units do not offer the facility. One of the oldest techniques is radioisotope imaging and intermittent reports still appear describing appearances in inflammatory myopathies; it is unlikely to achieve widespread usage. The most commonly used modalities are ultrasound, X-ray, computed tomography (CT) scanning, and magnetic resonance imaging (MRI). The information that can be gleaned from such studies is summarised in Table 2.10.

Table 2.10 *The principal uses of muscle imaging*

- Determining the distribution of muscle involvement
- Assessing the severity of muscle involvement
- Assessing disease progression
- Selecting a suitable muscle for biopsy

Clinically, the distribution of wasting and weakness may give a powerful clue as to the nature of the underlying disorder. Thus, neuropathies and the rare distal myopathies cause predominantly distal involvement, many myopathies have their onset in proximal muscles, and in many dystrophies there is highly selective involvement of certain muscles. Imaging may demonstrate such selectivity when it is not evident even to the most experienced clinical eye. One example is the demonstration of forearm flexor muscle disease in patients with inclusion body myositis prior to the clinical onset of the characteristic finger flexion weakness seen in this condition. Imaging may also give an indication of the severity of the disease process and can be used to assess disease progression or regression. Muscle bulk may be reduced. This tends to be more evident in neurogenic disorders, such as spinal muscular atrophy. In myopathic disorders muscle bulk tends to be preserved, despite weakness, and of course in the

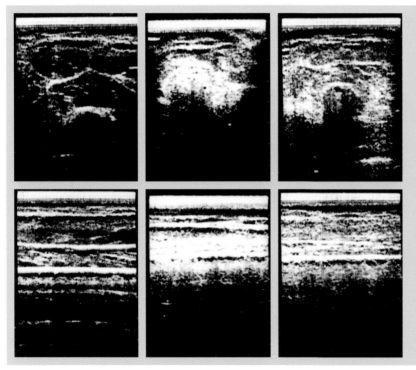

Figure 2.3 Muscle ultrasound scans. From a normal child, a child with spinal muscular atrophy, and one with limb-girdle muscular dystrophy. Note the increased echogenicity in the abnormal muscle. (Courtesy of Prof. Francesco Muntoni.)

dystrophies in particular one may see muscle hypertrophy. Imaging also shows fatty replacement in degenerating muscles. In many diseases not only is there selective muscle involvement but also the pathological changes may be patchy within a muscle. A consequence of this is the frustration of obtaining a normal muscle biopsy from an area of unaffected muscle. Ultrasound scanning has been found to be helpful, particularly in paediatric practice, in selecting an appropriate muscle for biopsy.

Ultrasound

Ultrasound has many obvious advantages over other imaging modalities; the equipment is portable and can be brought to the bedside, it is patient-friendly, the clinician can perform the study, and it is safe. Muscle bulk can be measured and pathological processes alter the muscles echogenicity (Figure 2.3). It is most useful in studying dystrophies and spinal muscular atrophy and, to a lesser extent, inflammatory myopathies. Findings are typically normal in metabolic myopathies. The value in selecting the muscle biopsy site was noted above.

X-ray computed tomography

Although CT has been the most widely described technique there is concern about the use of ionising radiation and it is likely to be supplanted by magnetic resonance imaging as the latter technique becomes more readily available. The generally accepted protocol involves transverse scans at several body levels, allowing assessment of a wide range of proximal and distal muscles. Muscle bulk is readily measured and density changes within muscle are defined in Hounsfield units. CT (and indeed MRI) is invaluable in identifying focal abnormalities such as cysts, abscesses and tumours.

Magnetic resonance imaging

Given its safety and sensitivity MRI is likely to become increasingly popular for investigating neuromuscular disorders but at present, in many parts of the world, it is a limited resource better put to other uses. As yet there have been few detailed reports of its use in a clinical setting but these are starting to appear. Selectivity of muscle involvement may be striking (Figure 2.4).

Biochemistry

In everyday practice the commonest muscle-oriented investigation is estimation of serum creatine kinase

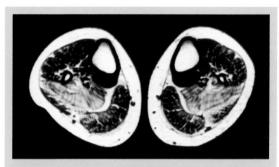

Figure 2.4 Muscle MRI scan. Calf scan in 16 year old ambulant girl with congenital muscular dystrophy. Note the selective involvement of soleus and relative sparing of tibialis anterior. (Courtesy of Prof. Francesco Muntoni.)

(CK). Many samples are sent for "routine biochemistry (i.e. liver function tests and electrolytes) and haematology", looking for adverse effects from immunosuppressive drugs used in treating inflammatory myopathies. In endocrine and acquired metabolic myopathies laboratory studies may of course be vital in establishing the diagnosis. Various forms of exercise testing, including phosphorus magnetic resonance spectroscopy, are helpful in diagnosing the rare inherited metabolic myopathies.

Blood and urine tests
Creatine kinase

By far and away the most useful investigation is estimation of serum creatine kinase (CK). The function of this enzyme is of no significance in the present context. Put simply, a wide range of muscle diseases damage muscle in such a way that CK contained within skeletal muscle is released into the circulation. Elevation of the serum CK is a non-specific marker of muscle disease or damage. As discussed below, some myopathies consistently cause profound elevation of the CK, others rarely cause an increase in CK, and there are many situations in which CK is elevated in the absence of neuromuscular disease. CK estimation is thus rather like neurophysiological studies - both may indicate the presence of muscle disease but neither is specific. Serial CK estimation can be helpful in monitoring disease progress but pitfalls exist. Unlike in general medicine, the various isoforms of CK are not of great importance and are rarely measured separately.

Table 2.11 indicates the typical change in serum CK level seen in a range of neuromuscular disorders. In

Table 2.11 Typical serum creatine kinase levels (CK) in a range of neuromuscular disorders*

Duchenne dystrophy	+++
Becker dystrophy	++ → +++
Emery–Dreifuss dystrophy	++
Limb-girdle dystrophies	N → +++
Congenital muscular dystrophy	+ → +++
Facioscapulohumeral dystrophy	N → +
Myotonic dystrophy	N → +
Distal myopathies	N → +++
Congenital (ultrastructural) myopathies	N → +
Idiopathic inflammatory myopathies	N → +++
Myotonia congenita	N → +
Periodic paralyses	N → +
Glycogenoses	+ → ++
Endocrine myopathies	N → + (except hypothyroidsm – can be ++)
Drug-induced	N → +++
Mitochondrial myopathies	N → +
Lipid-storage myopathies	N → ++
Spinal muscular atrophy/ motor neurone disease	N → +
Kennedy's syndrome	+ → ++

*Despite the use of international units (iu) different laboratories quote different "upper limits of normality". This table is based upon an upper limit of normal of 250 iu/l and the number of pluses indicates the following broad ranges:
+ = 250-1,000 iu/l
++ = 1,000-5,000 iu/l
+++ = > 5,000 iu/l
N = Normal

but there is an imprecise relationship between the level and muscle function. The CK typically falls to normal within weeks of starting corticosteroids but the weakness may take much longer to improve. Conversely, a rising CK level as steroids are reduced may be the first evidence of recurrence of disease activity. The CK is often normal in two of the commonest disorders seen in adults: myotonic dystrophy and facioscapulohumeral muscular dystrophy.

Elevation of the CK is seen in a number of settings in which there is clearly not a primary disorder of skeletal muscle, even though the muscles may be involved, and in which diagnostic confusion is not likely to arise - e.g. localised or generalised muscle trauma (including intramuscular injections, surgery, electric shock), sepsis, hypothermia, following intense or unaccustomed exercise, cardiac injury, with severe dyskinetic disorders and in acute psychosis. Much more important in clinical practice is the patient who is found to have an elevated CK level without obvious cause. Perhaps the commonest situation in which this arises is when a patient has "routine" blood tests and is found to have an elevated aspartate transaminase (AST) level. Despite the absence of other abnormal liver function tests, liver disease is often suspected and some patients go on to have a liver biopsy before it is realized that the AST is of skeletal muscle origin. When the penny drops the CK is estimated and found to be elevated. The commonest causes of an elevated CK in an otherwise apparently normal individual are shown in Table 2.12. Many patients have now been described who carry the Becker muscular dystrophy gene, and have an elevated CK level, but who do not have muscle weakness, at least at the time of presentation, are either asymptomatic or complain of exercise-induced myalgia and who may be susceptible to rhabdomyolysis.

Table 2.12 Causes of elevated creatine kinase (CK) in apparently normal individuals

- Hypothyroidism
- Becker muscular dystrophy
- Female carriers of the Duchenne/Becker muscular dystrophy gene
- Susceptibility to malignant hyperthermia
- Drugs causing sub-clinical myopathy (e.g. statins for treating hypercholesterolaemia)
- High level of physical exercise

Duchenne dystrophy the CK is invariably massively elevated in the early stages (and indeed heel-prick blood testing in neonates can be used as a reliable screening method) but falls later on as the muscle mass declines. Similarly, CK levels are typically very high in early cases of Becker dystrophy. Massive CK elevation is seen in acute rhabdomyolysis, which has many causes, including drug-induced. In the idiopathic inflammatory myopathies (dermatomyositis, polymyositis and inclusion body myositis) the CK is often but not always elevated. There is not always a correlation with the acuteness or severity. In chronic polymyositis with extensive weakness the CK can be normal. Also, in acute dermatomyositis it may be normal. If the CK is elevated then it may be used to help monitor progress,

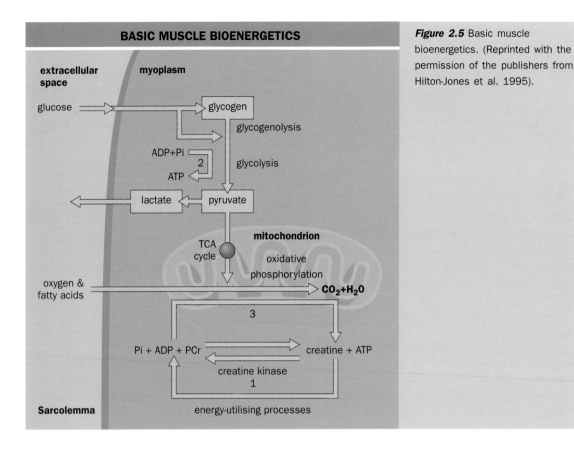

Figure 2.5 Basic muscle bioenergetics. (Reprinted with the permission of the publishers from Hilton-Jones et al. 1995).

Other biochemical tests

Although many other "muscle enzymes" can be assayed (e.g. myoglobin, aldolase, carbonic anhydrase III) none offers any particular advantage over CK and most routine laboratories reasonably refuse to do them. Urinary myoglobin is the cause of the very dark urine seen following an episode of acute rhabdomyolysis - it causes stick tests to give a positive result, which may cause confusion with haemoglobinuria. A specific myoglobin assay is available.

In mitochondrial disorders serum (and indeed CSF) lactate levels may be elevated in the resting state and these can be useful screening tests. Lactate and pyruvate levels are measured in the various exercise tests described below. In the relatively rare disorders of lipid metabolism blood and urine carnitine and acyl-carnitine assay are helpful. Diagnosis of these disorders is discussed elsewhere in this book.

Although useful as research tools, measurement of urinary protein metabolites such as creatine and 3-methylhistidine as indicators of muscle breakdown is rarely used in clinical practice.

Exercise tests

These are used in the investigation of suspected primary metabolic myopathies. Three types of test are commonly used. Forearm exercise testing and aerobic bicycle exercise are well established. They should only be performed at specialist centres by staff experienced in their use, partly because interpretation can be difficult and partly because they are not without hazard to the patient. Phosphorus magnetic resonance spectroscopy has proved very useful in the research setting but is available in only very few centres - it is unlikely to become more widely available. In many circumstances the diagnosis can readily be made without resorting to such investigations.

To understand the rationale behind these tests it is necessary to understand the basic principles of energy metabolism in muscle. Furthermore, this latter information is essential in understanding the symptomatology associated with specific disorders of muscle metabolism. The following section is an introduction to muscle bioenergetics and is followed by a brief description of each of the three main forms of exercise testing.

Muscle bioenergetics

The main energy requirement of muscle is for contraction, but energy is also required for other processes including re-uptake of calcium into the sarcoplasmic reticulum and the maintenance of concentration and electrochemical gradients. The immediate energy source within muscle is adenosine triphosphate (ATP) from which energy is released, in controlled fashion, during its enzymatic hydrolysis to adenosine diphosphate (ADP) and inorganic phosphate (Pi) (i.e. ATP $\rightarrow$ ADP + Pi). The amount of ATP stored in muscle is relatively small - a dozen or so forceful contractions would exhaust it. Muscle therefore depends on being able to re-synthesise ATP rapidly during exercise. Enzymatic defects in the various re-synthesis pathways lead to the primary, inherited, metabolic myopathies. The four pathways of particular importance are: creatine kinase reaction; glycolysis; oxidative phosphorylation; and adenylate kinase and myoadenylate deaminase (Figure 2.5).

Creatine kinase reaction

At the onset of exercise the major energy generating pathways of glycolysis and oxidative phosphorylation, described below, have not had time to become activated. The immediate, but very limited, source of ATP repletion is the creatine kinase reaction (i.e. phosphocreatine (PCr) + ADP + H+ $\leftrightarrow$ Creatine + ATP). This reaction is of particular importance in understanding and interpreting phosphorus magnetic resonance spectroscopy data.

Glycolysis

Blood glucose is not generally an important direct energy source in muscle. Rather, glucose entering muscle fibres is stored, for future use, as glycogen. Whether derived directly from glucose or from glycogen, the starting point of glycolysis is glucose-6-phosphate (Figure 2.6). The pathway from glucose-6-phosphate to pyruvate generates ATP anaerobically. In

Figure 2.6 The pathways of glycogen synthesis and breakdown (glycogenolysis) and of glycolysis. Enzymes known to be associated with deficiency states are shown in bold print. The sites of NAD⁺, NADH, ADP and ADP utilisation and production are indicated. (Reprinted with the permission of the publishers from Hilton-Jones et al. 1995).

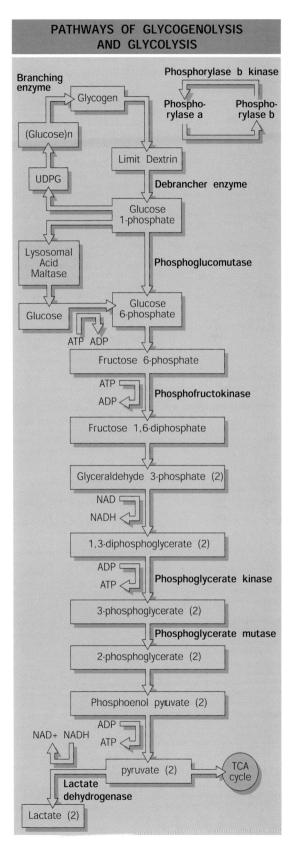

PATHWAYS OF GLYCOGENOLYSIS AND GLYCOLYSIS

the presence of an adequate oxygen supply the pyruvate is oxidised in the mitochondria, via Krebs' cycle and the electron transport chain, with the generation of considerably more ATP than is available from glycolysis. In the absence of sufficient oxygen pyruvate is reduced to lactate.

Oxidative phosphorylation

This term describes the process by which ATP is synthesised from ADP as a result of the transfer of electrons from NADH (reduced nicotinamide adenine dinucleotide) and FADH2 (reduced flavine adenine dinucleotide) to molecular oxygen by a series of electron carriers (the respiratory chain) located in the inner mitochondrial membrane. NADH and FADH2 are energy-rich molecules formed during glycolysis, fatty acid oxidation and Krebs' (tri-carboxylic acid) cycle. Oxidative phosphorylation is thus dependent upon an adequate supply of substrates and oxygen to muscle which, as discussed below, is not always the case in certain stages of exercise.

Adenylate kinase and myoadenylate deaminase

Although the adenylate kinase and myoadenylate deaminase reactions (Figure 2.7) are quantitatively unimportant in terms of ATP generation, they result in the production of ammonia. Estimation of ammonia generation is an essential part of the forearm exercise test (see below).

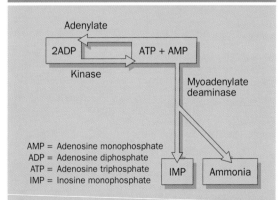

Figure 2.7 The adenylate kinase and myoadenylate kinase reactions.
AMP = Adenosine monophosphate
ADP = Adenosine diphosphate
ATP = Adenosine triphosphate
IMP = Inosine monophosphate

Metabolic changes during exercise

At rest the energetic demand of skeletal muscle is modest and is met entirely through the oxidation of fatty acids. That is, the blood supply to the muscle delivers adequate amounts of free fatty acids and oxygen. The fatty acids undergo β-oxidation within mitochondria generating acetyl-CoA, which enters Krebs' cycle, and the electron donors NADH and FADH2. Initiation of exercise leads to an immediate increase in ATP utilisation. With vigorous exercise the energy demand may increase by several orders of magnitude. Oxidative metabolism cannot cope because in the early stages of exercise there is insufficient delivery of substrate (e.g. fatty acids) and oxygen. The immediate source of ATP, although of very limited capacity, is the creatine kinase reaction. Within a few seconds glycolysis is activated. Glucose moieties are released from the glycogen stored in muscle and the glycolytic pathway results in the production of ATP and pyruvate (Figures 2.5 & 2.6). Because of the limited availability of oxygen, pyruvate is reduced to lactate rather than being oxidised in the mitochondria. Lactate diffuses out of the muscle and enters the circulation. In addition, the rise in ADP concentration as a result of ATP hydrolysis results in the generation of ammonia through the adenylate kinase and myoadenylate deaminase pathways (Figure 2.7). The measurement of lactate and ammonia forms the basis of the forearm exercise test (see below).

As exercise continues adaptive processes take place. Blood flow to muscle increases, the respiratory rate increases and free fatty acids enter the circulation from the body's lipid stores. Glycogen stores within muscle become depleted. Thus with sustained activity muscle metabolism switches back from being predominantly anaerobic at the start of exercise to being predominantly aerobic; lactate levels fall as more and more pyruvate can be dealt with via Krebs' cycle and at the same time free fatty acid levels in the blood increase.

At a first approximation the clinical features of the major metabolic myopathies can be understood in terms of the biochemical processes described above. The glycogen storage disorders (e.g. myophosphorylase deficiency) are most likely to cause symptoms at the start of exercise, particularly if intense, because that is when muscle is most dependent upon glycolysis. Indeed, patients complain of pain, weakness and cramp in just these circumstances. If they continue to exercise, their symptoms ease as oxidative metabolism becomes increasingly important to ATP generation (the so-called "second-wind" phenomenon). At rest, when glycolysis is inactive, one might expect no symptoms

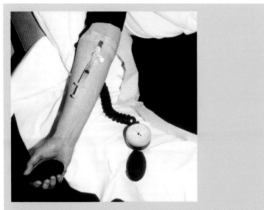

Figure 2.8 The ischaemic forearm exercise test. Note the cannula, arm cuff and sphygmomanometer bulb. Although the traditional approach, it is preferable to perform the test without arterial occlusion (see text).

but, although that is often the case, glycogen accumulation can interfere with muscle fibre function such that the patient has permanent weakness. Disorders of fatty acid metabolism or of the respiratory chain, insufficient to compromise the relatively minor metabolic requirements of muscle at rest, might be expected to produce symptoms on sustained exercise. That is indeed the case and for several such disorders the classical presentation is during long route-marches.

Forearm exercise test

The forearm exercise test is a relatively simple test used to screen for defects of glycogenolysis and glycolysis (Figure 2.6); the biochemical basis is discussed above. Originally, and as described below, the test was performed ischaemically, by occluding blood supply to the forearm during exercise. The test is not without hazard (rhabdomyolysis, occasionally severe enough to affect renal function, can occur) and should only be done by a team with appropriate expertise. In part because of this concern, and noting that oxidative metabolism contributes little in the early stages of intense exercise, some units prefer to perform the test without inducing ischaemia.

A plastic cannula (with tap attached and kept patent with the use of heparin) is inserted into the median cubital vein (Figure 2.8). This should be done with minimum venous stasis and 15 minutes or more before the start of the test proper. A base-line blood sample is taken and then the forearm made ischaemic by inflating an arm cuff to above arterial blood pressure. The patient then exercises the forearm flexor muscles by repeatedly squeezing a sphygmomanometer bulb to the point of exhaustion,

which takes between one and two minutes. The arm cuff is then released and further blood samples are taken, typically immediately and at 1, 2, 3, 5, 10, 15 and 20 minutes after release of the cuff. Each sample is assayed for lactate and ammonia (special sample bottles and rapid processing are required, so the test must be done in close collaboration with the biochemistry laboratory).

The normal response is an increase over baseline levels of both venous lactate and ammonia. In disorders of glycogenolysis and glycolysis the lactate response is sub-normal or absent and the rise in ammonia excessive. Conversely, in myoadenylate deaminase deficiency there is a normal rise in lactate but little or no increase in ammonia. If the patient simply does not exercise the forearm flexor muscles enough (a not uncommon experience in patients with non-organic muscle symptomatology such as fatigue and myalgia) then neither the lactate nor the ammonia levels increase. Each laboratory must determine its own normal ranges for the changes in lactate and ammonia.

There are many ways in which the results can be expressed. If the maximum change in lactate level is plotted against the maximum change in ammonia, then it is possible to discriminate between normal individuals, those with glycogenolytic/glycolytic defects and those with myoadenylate deaminase deficiency. This is illustrated in Figure 2.9, but

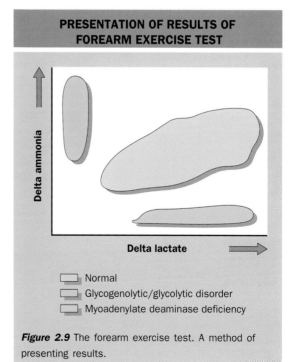

PRESENTATION OF RESULTS OF FOREARM EXERCISE TEST

Delta ammonia

Delta lactate

☐ Normal
☐ Glycogenolytic/glycolytic disorder
☐ Myoadenylate deaminase deficiency

Figure 2.9 The forearm exercise test. A method of presenting results.

without absolute values being given, because these must be determined by individual laboratories.

Aerobic bicycle exercise test

There is a long history of the use of static bicycle exercise and the measurement of associated metabolic changes in the study of normal exercise physiology. In clinical practice the main value of the technique is in the investigation of patients suspected of having a disorder of oxidative metabolism, most notably the mitochondrial cytopathies. Normally, as noted above, pyruvate is metabolised via Krebs' cycle and the respiratory chain. If there is a defect in this pathway then pyruvate is reduced to lactate. In the test, the patient exercises, typically for 15 minutes, and lactate (and sometimes pyruvate) is measured during exercise and recovery. Many protocols have been described, the main difficulty being to quantitate the level of exercise. The most satisfactory is the so-called sub-anaerobic threshold exercise test. In disorders of oxidative metabolism there is an abnormal increase in the level of lactate and also an abnormal lactate/pyruvate ratio. Each laboratory must establish its own confidence limits.

Phosphorus magnetic resonance spectroscopy

All clinicians are nowadays familiar with magnetic resonance imaging, which depends upon the magnetic properties of tissue protons. Although much less widely available phosphorus magnetic resonance spectroscopy has contributed significantly to our understanding of a number of myopathies and in those few centres where it is available it is a useful diagnostic tool, particularly in the study of metabolic myopathies. Although proton imaging can be performed at a relatively low magnetic field strength, phosphorus spectroscopy requires a magnet of at least 1.5 Tesla.

The position of a phosphorus nucleus within a molecule affects its resonant frequency, allowing us to identify different phosphorus-containing metabolites (Figure 2.10). Under appropriate conditions it can be shown that the signal intensity is proportional to concentration. It is fortunate for us that the technique identifies compounds that are of such major importance with respect to muscle bioenergetics. ATP produces three peaks because each of its three phosphorus nuclei is in a different chemical environment. Because it is bound, and only unbound molecules give rise to distinct peaks, ADP is not detected, but its concentration can be calculated from

the creatine kinase equilibrium expression: *phosphocreatine + ADP + H+ → Creatine + ATP*.

As noted, signal intensity is proportional to metabolite concentration and thus from the spectra concentration ratios can be determined. If the true concentration of one metabolite is known (in practice, the concentration of ATP measured by direct assay on biopsy samples is used) then absolute concentrations of other metabolites, including ADP, can be derived. The phosphomonoester peak is derived from a number of metabolites, including the phosphorylated intermediates of glycolysis. Information about the metabolic status of the muscle can be obtained at rest, during exercise, and during recovery.

The resting spectrum may be abnormal in mitochondrial disorders (Figure 2.10), even in the absence of histological changes. The ratios Pi/ATP and Pi/PCr may be increased, and PCr/ATP decreased, as a result of a decrease in PCr concentration and increase in Pi concentration. The calculated ADP concentration is reduced, leading to a reduction in the phosphorylation potential ([ATP]/[ADP][Pi]) which is a measure of the amount of energy available.

During exercise PCr concentration falls as it is utilized to generate ATP. Glycolysis becomes active and pH falls as a result of lactic acid generation. In mitochondrial, glycogenolytic and glycolytic disorders, all of which limit ATP generation, the rate of fall of PCr is greater than normal. In mitochondrial disorders glycogenolysis and glycolysis are enhanced and it can be shown that proton production is greater than normal. Conversely, in disorders of glycogenolysis and glycolysis (Figure 2.6) lactate production is impaired and pH does not fall - in fact, it tends to rise as the breakdown of phosphocreatine in the creatine kinase reaction, shown above, is associated with proton consumption. With disorders of the lower part of the glycolytic pathway, such as phosphoglycerate mutase deficiency (Figure 2.6), the phosphorylated intermediates of glycolysis accumulate and give rise to an enhanced phosphomonoester peak (Figure 2.10). It can be seen that an exercise phosphorus spectroscopy study, which is performed aerobically, can give similar information to the conventional forearm exercise test described above. Failure of lactate generation is shown by absence of a fall in pH. Instead of a rise in ammonia, the fall in PCr shows that the subject is making sufficient effort. Accumulation of phosphomonoesters suggests a defect of the more distal part of the pathway, rather than a more proximal defect such as debrancher enzyme or myophosphorylase deficiency.

Metabolic recovery following exercise is an entirely oxidative process and phosphorus spectroscopy data during recovery act as a sensitive indicator of mitochondrial dysfunction. The most useful measure is the rate of PCr recovery. PCr recovery is also slower with defects of distal glycolysis due to trapping of Pi, which is required for PCr regeneration, in the phosphorylated intermediates.

PHOSPHORUS MAGNETIC RESONANCE SPECTROSCOPY

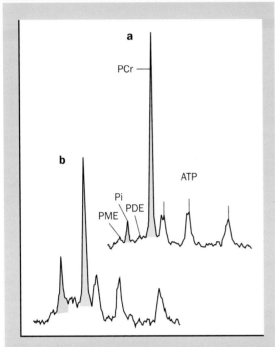

PCr = Phosphocreatine
Pi = Inorganic phosphate
ATP = Adenosine triphosphate
PME = Phosphomonoesters
PDE = Phosphodiesters

Figure 2.10 Phosphorus magnetic resonance spectroscopy. Spectra of resting gastrocnemius muscle from a normal control subject (a) and a patient with mitochondrial myopathy (b) are shown. The x-axis represents chemical shift (or resonance frequency) and the y-axis signal intensity, which under certain conditions also reflects concentration.

PCr = phosphocreatine
Pi   = inorganic phosphate
ATP = adenosine triphosphate
PME = phosphomonoesters
PDE = phosphodiesters

pH can be determined from the chemical shift between the Pi and PCr signals; it is 7.03 in (a) and 7.10 in (b). (Reproduced with permission from the publishers from Hilton-Jones et al. 1995.)

Enzyme assay

In many of the metabolic myopathies the diagnosis is secured by enzyme assay. This will often be performed on a muscle biopsy specimen and as a general rule a sample should be frozen and stored (at -70°C) whenever a biopsy is taken (apart from metabolic myopathies, such material may be used at a later date for protein studies as new causes of muscular dystrophies are identified). In some disorders assays may be performed on blood, urine, fibroblast cultures, and liver biopsy specimens.

Muscle biopsy

Despite the rapid evolution in genetics and molecular biology, muscle biopsy remains the single most important diagnostic tool when considering primary disorders of muscle. It is of less value in studying neurogenic disorders although it may be the appearances on biopsy that first point towards a neurogenic rather than myopathic process. As with electromyography it must be remembered that taken alone biopsy results may be misleading. So-called secondary myopathic changes may be seen in some chronic neurogenic disorders. Furthermore, pathological changes may be very focal, both within a particular muscle and between muscles. This is particularly well recognised in idiopathic inflammatory myopathies in which a first biopsy may show no abnormality and a second rampant changes. It is often helpful in such cases to sample multiple levels through the specimen. That a single biopsy may not be representative of the underlying pathological process is emphasised in Figure 2.11. Biopsy appearances in specific disorders are considered throughout this book and this section provides only a broad overview of biopsy techniques, histological methods and findings. There are several excellent monographs on muscle biopsy (e.g. Carpenter and Karpati 2000; Dubowitz 1985) and Dubowitz provides a useful guide on "How to read a biopsy". It is our view that a close collaboration between clinician and pathologist is essential to get the maximum information from muscle biopsies.

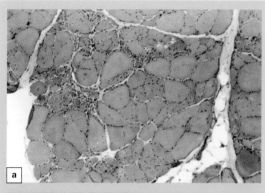
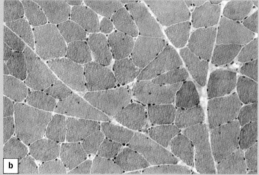

Figure 2.11 Biopsy findings may be unrepresentative. Two muscle biopsy samples from the same patient (a 60 year old male with an unusual form of rigid spine syndrome). The first sample (a), from vastus lateralis, showed extensive pathological changes. A further biopsy was performed in order to obtain additional material for protein studies. The second, (b), from deltoid, showed only a few atrophic fibres. Both muscles were affected clinically.

The biopsy procedure

Which muscle is chosen for biopsy will to some extent depend upon the experience of the person performing the biopsy and which biopsy technique is being used. Open biopsies are generally performed on one of a few muscles, the commonest being deltoid and vastus lateralis (quadriceps). With needle biopsy many other muscles can safely be biopsied. The muscle chosen should be mildly to moderately weak to give the best chance of identifying specific pathological features. In severely weak muscles the microscopic appearance is often that of "end-stage" muscle, with extensive replacement of muscle fibres by fat and connective tissue and any earlier specific pathological changes have been lost.

Open biopsy and needle biopsy each have their proponents. Both are performed using local anaesthesia and there are very few indications for biopsy under general anaesthesia, which is unsafe in a number of myopathies. Needle biopsy involves a smaller incision and thus less scarring, but the sample is small, causing problems with handling and orientation, and as noted above, in patchy disorders, pathological changes may be missed. Repeat samples can be taken and the method has been used widely in physiological research. Open biopsies are more invasive but the operator can see the muscle being sampled and can avoid tendon insertion sites. The specimen is readily orientated and multiple levels can be examined. Adequate specimens for biochemical studies can be obtained. Broadly speaking, needle biopsy is favoured in paediatric practice and open biopsy for adults.

The surgeon should have adequate experience. In many centres the operator is either the pathologist who reads the specimen or the neuromuscular clinician responsible for the patient. Specimen preparation differs considerably from routine processing of surgical specimens (which typically involves formalin fixation and wax embedding – methods that are of little value in the study of muscle diseases) and should only be done in a laboratory with appropriate experience.

Specimen handling and assessment

Apart from the specimen for microscopic study, a sample should be frozen in liquid nitrogen for future biochemical and DNA analysis, and another fixed for semi-thin sections and electron microscopy. In certain circumstances a piece of muscle may be put in culture medium for the establishment of cell lines.

The specimen for light microscopy is orientated under a dissecting microscope, fixed on a cork disc, and then snap frozen by immersion in cooled isopentane. Sections (6μm tick) are cut on a cryostat and mounted on glass coverslips, ready for staining.

Histology and histochemistry

A panel of routine histological and histochemical stains (Table 2.13) are applied to each biopsy specimen. Additional stains may be used in specific circumstances, such as myophosphorylase staining in suspected McArdle's disease.

Immunocytochemistry (ICC)

In this method biopsy sections are incubated with an antibody directed against a specific antigen. The antibody is labelled with a coloured tag that can be visualised either by direct light microscopy or which fluoresces under ultra-violet light. Thus, the antigen can be identified and localised. Its widest use is found in the study of muscular dystrophies and inflammatory

Table 2.13. *Routine muscle biopsy techniques and their uses*

Tissue dyes	Uses
Haematoxylin and eosin	Routine histology
Gomori's modified trichrome	Routine histology
Periodic acid-Schiff	Identifying excess glycogen
Oil red O	Identifying excess lipid
Histochemistry	**Uses**
ATPase (pH 9.4, 4.6 and 4.3)	Fibre typing
NADH-TR*	Myofibrillar organization
Succinate dehydrogenase	Assessing mitochondrial number and distribution
Cytochrome oxidase	Assessing mitochondrial distribution and function
Acid phosphatase	Assessing lysosomal activity and identifying macrophages

myopathies. It can also be used to label enzymes in suspected metabolic myopathies but care must be taken because the presence of antigenically active enzyme does not necessarily mean that it is functionally active.

Electron microscopy (EM)

EM has taught us a great deal about the ultra-structure of muscle in both health and disease. It is time consuming and therefore perhaps fortunately is not used routinely in clinical practice, but rather is applied to a few specific clinical problems. In adults its main role is in the identification of filamentous inclusions in inclusion body myositis and oculopharyngeal muscular dystrophy, and in children in the characterisation of ultra-structural abnormalities in a variety of congenital myopathies.

Major pathological features

The following is a brief summary of the main pathological features seen in some of the commoner neuromuscular disorders.

Denervation

The exact appearance depends upon the chronicity of the underlying neurogenic problem. Features include small angular fibres, which may occur in groups (particularly in anterior horn cell disorders), and in more chronic disorders fibre-type grouping (Figure 2.12). Such groups, in which all of the fibres are of the same histochemical type (as identified by ATPase staining), reflect reinnervation by collateral sprouting from the terminal axons of surviving neurones.

Muscular dystrophies

In Duchenne muscular dystrophy (Figure 2.13) the characteristic features, none of which are specific to this particular disorder, include fibre necrosis and phagocytosis, regenerating fibres, many rounded fibres (including hypercontracted hyaline or opaque fibres), and extensive replacement by connective tissue. In Becker and other limb-girdle dystrophies the appearances are usually less severe. There is an increase in

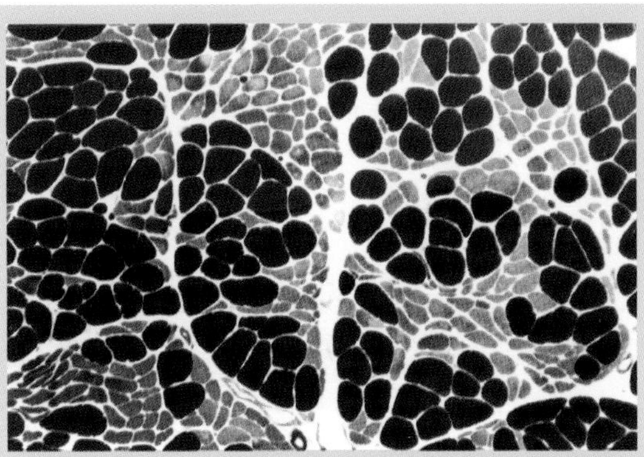

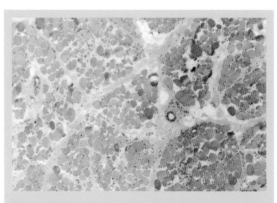

Figure 2.12 Denervation and reinnervation. Myosin ATPase (pH 9.6). See text for explanation.

Figure 2.13 Duchenne muscular dystrophy. See text for discussion.

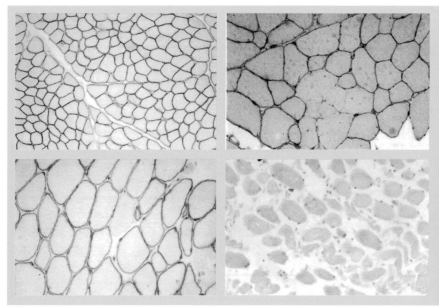

Figure 2.14 Dystrophin immunocytochemistry. Normal – (top left) – note even staining around periphery of each fibre. Duchenne dystrophy – (bottom right) – note complete absence of dystrophin staining. Becker dystrophy – (bottom left) – note irregular staining around the periphery, and occasional fibres showing no staining. Female Duchenne carrier – (top right) – note cluster of negatively staining fibres.

the normal variability of fibre size, a variable degree of necrosis, splitting of fibres, increased numbers of internal nuclei, and increased fibrous tissue.

Immunocytochemistry (Figure 2.14) shows that dystrophin is absent in Duchenne dystrophy. In Becker dystrophy the dystrophin staining may be irregular around individual fibres and between fibres, but it may appear normal and Western blotting is required to show reduced levels of dystrophin or the presence of a protein with reduced molecular weight. In manifesting female carriers individual fibres may show variable or absent dystrophin expression. Immunocytochemical methods for other forms of limb-girdle muscular dystrophy are evolving rapidly and are discussed in more detail in Chapter 4.

In facioscapulohumeral and myotonic dystrophy, the commonest dystrophies seen in adults, there are no specific biopsy features and biopsy does not form part of their routine assessment. Characteristic filaments are seen on biopsy in oculopharyngeal muscular dystrophy, but this diagnosis is now made by DNA analysis.

Congenital myopathies

Congenital myopathies comprise a number of unrelated disorders which show different features on muscle biopsy. Some of these are characterised by ultra-structural abnormalities and indeed they are sometimes called the ultra-structural myopathies. In some the muscle fibre architecture is deranged (e.g. central core disease, multicore disease, centronuclear

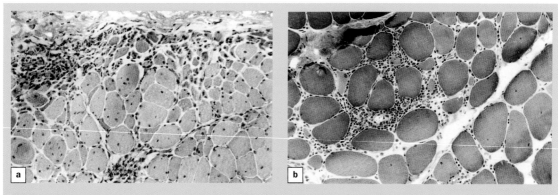

Figure 2.15 (a) Dermatomyositis – inflammatory infiltrate concentrated around blood vessels. (b) Polymyositis – perimysial distribution of inflammatory infiltrate.

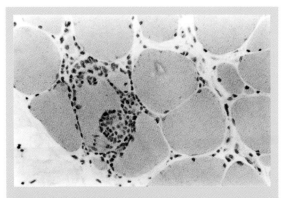

Figure 2.16 Partial invasion. Lymphocytes are invading a non-necrotic muscle fibre. (Polymyositis).

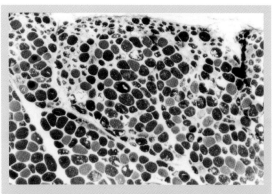

Figure 2.17 Perifascicular atrophy in dermatomyositis.

myopathy). In others there are abnormal structures or accumulations within fibres (e.g. nemaline myopathy, desmin-storage myopathies, fingerprint body myopathy), and in others there is an abnormality of organelles (e.g. tubular aggregate myopathy).

Inflammatory myopathies

The characteristic feature of the idiopathic inflammatory myopathies (dermatomyositis, polymyositis, inclusion body myositis) is the presence of inflammatory infiltrates (Figure 2.15) composed mainly of lymphocytes and some macrophages. In dermatomyositis (DM) the infiltrates tend to be perivascular and immunocytochemistry shows that B-cells predominate over T-cells, and that amongst the T-cells helper types (T4+, CD4) predominate over cytotoxic cells (T8+, CD8). Conversely, in polymyositis (PM) and inclusion body myositis (IBM) the infiltrates tend to be scattered within fascicles with T-lymphocytes (predominantly T8+) being more numerous than B-cells. In PM and IBM clusters of inflammatory cells may be seen apparently compressing or indenting a non-necrotic muscle fibre - a phenomenon known as partial invasion (Figure 2.16).

In dermatomyositis capillary numbers are reduced. Necrotic fibres may be seen in isolation, or in groups secondary to infarction. Perifascicular atrophy may be striking (Figure 2.17). In polymyositis and inclusion body myositis necrotic fibres are scattered throughout the fascicles.

Metabolic myopathies

Muscle biopsy appearances in metabolic myopathies have been reviewed. Necrosis and regeneration are generally not prominent features except after an acute

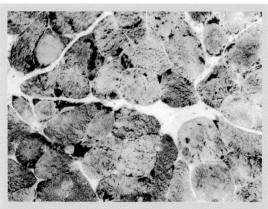

Figure 2.18 Glycogen accumulation in debrancher enzyme deficiency (PAS stain).

episode of muscle damage following a metabolic crisis, for example brought on by intense exercise.

Glycogenolytic/glycolytic disorder

Excess glycogen storage is readily seen using the periodic acid-Schiff (PAS) stain. It is often striking in the more proximal glycogenolytic/glycolytic disorders such as debrancher enzyme deficiency (Figure 2.18), but with defects involving the more distal part of the glycolytic pathway (Figure 2.6) it is typically absent, presumably because alternative pathways exist. The glycogen lies free between myofibrils and may form large lakes. In acid maltase deficiency the excess glycogen is contained within lysosomes.

Excessive lipid storage is seen in a number of myopathies associated with disordered lipid metabolism but it is by no means invariable. In carnitine

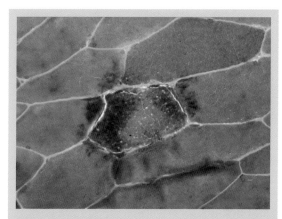

Figure 2.19 Ragged red fibres (modified Gomori trichrome).

palmitoyltransferase deficiency the biopsy usually appears normal, but there may be some excess lipid following an acute episode.

Mitochondrial cytopathies
A characteristic feature of mitochondrial cytopathies is the presence of ragged red fibres, seen using the modified Gomori trichrome stain (Figure 2.19). Mitochondria stain red and the appearance is due to aggregations of mitochondria within fibres and particularly in the sub-sarcolemmal region. Such fibres also appear abnormal with haematoxylin and eosin, succinate dehydrogenase, and NADH staining. The cytochrome oxidase (COX) stain may show mitochondrial collections, but in addition in some mitochondrial cytopathies a characteristic feature is the presence of COX-negative fibres, reflecting impaired enzyme activity. Although not essential for diagnosis, electron microscopy shows accumulations of structurally abnormal mitochondria, which may also contain paracrystalline inclusions.

Molecular diagnosis

The methods of molecular biology are advancing so rapidly that many of the comments made in this book about the molecular basis of specific disorders will be out of date long before the book reaches the sellers shelves. The rate of development is so rapid that the most effective way of keeping up to date is by reference to internet websites that detail genotype data (e.g. the Cambridge site recording mutations in Emery-Dreifuss dystrophy at http://www.path.cam.ac.

uk/emd/). Specific details about individual disorders will be made in the appropriate chapters. However, it is possible to make some general comments.

The single most important technique has been that of positional cloning (also called "reverse genetics"). What might be called conventional methods relied upon identification of the defective protein and then tracing backwards to find the mutated gene. The problem in many disorders is/was that the defective protein is/was unknown. Positional cloning allows identification of the gene and then of the protein product. The commonest approach is through the study of large informative families with a clinically clearly defined disorder. By the use of polymorphic markers the chromosomal position of the gene is identified. The exact position of the gene is determined by using finer mapping techniques. Expressed transcripts from the area are assessed as possible candidate genes. Once the gene is identified the protein product can be deduced from the nucleotide sequence, which of course determines the amino acid sequence.

Another important approach is by studying candidate genes. The Human Genome Project has led to identification of all genes. Specific pathophysiological or biochemical features of a disorder might suggest the type of protein that is abnormal. Relevant candidate genes can then be screened to look for associated mutations.

The identification of the gene defect causing a particular disorder is likely to be a major prerequisite to the development of effective therapy, whether this be by "genetic engineering" or by biochemical means. This is for the future, but there are immediate practical benefits to the patient and their family of having a specific genetic diagnosis (Table 2.14). Most of these benefits are self-evident and specific aspects will be

Table 2.14 *Advantages to patient and family of identifying a specific disease-causing gene abnormality*

- DNA studies
- Precise diagnosis
- Carrier identification
- Identification of pre-symptomatic individuals
- Accurate genetic counselling
- Pre-natal diagnosis possible
- Occasionally, prediction of phenotype and severity

Table 2.15 *The types of gene mutation seen in the commoner neuromuscular disorders*

Large deletions	Duchenne/Becker muscular dystrophy (most patients)
Small deletions & point mutations	Duchenne/Becker muscular dystrophy (up to 30%)
Deletion	Spinal muscular atrophy
	Mitochondrial cytopathies (especially chronic external ophthalmoplegia) – in mitochondrial DNA
	Hereditary liability to pressure palsies
Duplication	Hereditary motor and sensory neuropathy IA
Point mutations	Sarcoglycanopathies
	Limb girdle dystrophy 2A (calpain-deficient)
	Congenital muscular dystrophy (merosin deficient)
	Many metabolic disorders
	Channelopathies
	Myotonia congenita
	Emery-Dreifuss X-linked muscular dystrophy
	Hereditary motor and sensory neuropathy (several)
	Mitochondrial cytopathies (in mitochondrial DNA)
	Congenital myasthenic syndromes
Trinucleotide repeat expansion	Myotonic dystrophy
	Kennedy's syndrome
	Oculopharyngeal muscular dystrophy
Deletion of repeat units	Facioscapulohumeral muscular dystrophy

considered when discussing individual disorders. With respect to identification of carriers and pre-symptomatic individuals it is particularly important to consider those diseases in which the offspring may be more severely affected than the parent. This is clearly the case for X-linked disorders. Female carriers of the Duchenne/Becker gene and the Emery-Dreifuss gene are usually (but not always) asymptomatic but their sons may be affected. Perhaps less well appreciated is the situation seen in myotonic dystrophy (and some other gene-expansion disorders) when a severely affected child is born to an asymptomatic or oligosymptomatic mother, who may or may not later develop obvious features of the disease.

Several different types of mutation are seen in neuromuscular disorders. These are summarised, for the more commonly encountered nerve and muscle disorders, in Table 2.15.

Ancillary investigations

Many muscle disorders are part of a multi-system disease process (see Chapter 1). Investigations other than those directed specifically at muscle may serve several purposes. A particular pattern of multi-system involvement may point to a specific diagnosis - for example, the combination of skeletal muscle and liver disease in some of the glycogenoses. In some conditions it may not be the muscle disorder that presents the major threat with respect to morbidity and mortality. Thus, it is important to identify cardiac disease, which is often sub-clinical, in patients with dystrophinopathy, Emery-Dreifuss syndrome and myotonic dystrophy. Similarly, respiratory muscle involvement causing ventilatory insufficiency may be seen even in the presence of minimal skeletal muscle dysfunction in acid maltase deficiency, motor neurone disease and various forms of rigid spine syndrome.

Depending on the primary diagnosis, consideration may have to be given to investigating the heart (ECG and echocardiography), central nervous system (MRI, evoked potential studies, audiometry, electroencephalography, neuropsychological assessment), peripheral nerves (nerve conduction studies), respiratory function (vital capacity, sleep apnoea), haematological parameters, and liver, kidney and endocrine function.

Selected further reading

Carpenter S, Karpati G. *Pathology of Skeletal Muscle*. New York: Oxford University Press Inc, 2000.

Coleman RA, Stajich JM, Pact VW, Pericak-Vance MA. Ischemic exercise test in normal adults and in patients with weakness and cramps. *Muscle Nerve* 1986; 9: 216–221

De Visser M, Reimers CD. Muscle imaging. In: Engel AG, Franzini-Armstrong C (eds). *Myology* 2nd edn. New York: McGraw-Hill, 1994: 795-806.

Dubowitz V. *Muscle Biopsy. A practical approach* 2nd edn. London: Baillière Tindall, 1985.

Dubowitz V. *Muscle Disorders in Childhood* 2nd edn. London: Saunders, 1995.

Engel AG, Franzini-Armstrong C (eds). *Myology* 2nd edn. New York: McGraw-Hill, 1994.

Haller RG, Bertocci LA (1994). Exercise evaluation of metabolic myopathies. In: Engel AG, Franzini-Armstrong C (eds). *Myology* 2nd edn. New York: McGraw-Hill, 1994: 807–821.

Hilton-Jones D, Squier M, Taylor D, Matthews P (eds). *Metabolic Myopathies*. London: WB Saunders, 1995.

Karpati G, Hilton-Jones D, Griggs R (eds). *Disorders of Voluntary Muscle* 7th edn. Cambridge: Cambridge University Press, 2001.

Kimura J (1989) *Electrodiagnosis in diseases of nerve and muscle* 2nd edn. Philadelphia: FA Davis, 1989.

Lane RJM (ed). *Handbook of Muscle Disease*. New York: Marcel Dekker, 1996.

Nashef L, Lane RJM. Screening for mitochondrial cytopathies: the sub-anaerobic threshold exercise test (SATET). *J Neurol Neurosurg Psych* 1989; 52: 1090–1094

Sinkeler SP, Wevers RA, Joosten EM et al. Improvement of screening in exertional myalgia with a standardized ischemic forearm test. *Muscle Nerve* 1986; 9: 731–737.

Swash M, Brown MM, Thakkar C. CT muscle imaging and the clinical assessment of neuromuscular disease. *Muscle Nerve* 1995; 18: 708–714

chapter 3

Principles of therapy
of neuromuscular disease

Introduction

All too often the clinician making a diagnosis of neuro-muscular disease is of the opinion that, once the diagnosis is made, there is nothing more he or she can do. The patient or their family will be given a name for their disease, an idea that it may be inherited and the information that it is incurable and is likely to slowly get worse. If the patient is lucky the address of a support organisation may be offered. Follow up may be considered if the clinic is not too busy, but often only to have "teaching material" for medical education. Not surprisingly the patient and their family are often devastated. The idea that failure to cure or slow a disease with medication means that there is "nothing that I can do for you" is a sad reflection on the lack of a holistic or rehabilitative approach from the clinicians involved.

In this chapter we will show that holistic therapy for these patients is possible and includes careful handling at the time of diagnosis, the identification and treatment of those diseases for which drug therapy is possible as well as the recognition, and wherever possible, prevention of avoidable and predictable co-morbidity.

The time of diagnosis

Whenever possible a clear and accurate diagnosis must be made. For example, the treatment of patients with adult-onset myopathies and an "irritable" EMG with corticosteroids on the grounds that they might have polymyositis is not good practice any more than the diagnosis and treatment of lung cancer purely by means of a chest X-ray. Where diagnosis can be made non-invasively, as with genetic testing in many cases of Duchenne or Becker muscular dystrophy, then biopsy can be avoided without loss of diagnostic accuracy. In other cases invasive testing is needed and the patient or family need to be beware of the importance of diagnostic precision. Where there is a strong suspicion of a particular disease or disease-type then this may be gently introduced to the patient in the form of part of a differential diagnosis before a definitive diagnosis is made. The final diagnosis is often then less of a shock and many patients will have sensible questions to ask when the definitive diagnosis is first announced. The patient or parents may have a specific fear about one diagnosis and to hear that you are considering it will mean they know you are taking their fears seriously. Where there is not such a firm diagnostic possibility one should talk in more general terms rather than to introduce unnecessary fears to the patients.

When diagnosing inflammatory myopathies or myasthenia the news is often relatively good, since the patient is presented with a good chance of significant functional recovery or even cure. Similarly some other patients may be reassured that they have a non-progressive and benign disorder such as myotonia congenita, and that symptomatic treatments are available.

For others, however, the time of diagnosis may be a grim and unwelcome time when their worst fears are confirmed. There is no simple recipe for how to handle this situation. It is well established that patients assimilate only 10% or so of information given in a medical consultation. At a time of great shock even less will be remembered. It is thus best to keep things as simple and straightforward as possible and to emphasise that there is much that can be done in terms of support, without dwelling upon specifics (Table 3.1). Written information may be very helpful and patients should be put in touch with their local or national support group or charity, such as the Muscular Dystrophy Campaign, or the Muscular Dystrophy Association in the USA. If more information is sought then it should be given honestly but sensitively. Questions about prognosis are particularly difficult. The patient may ask without really wanting to know, and relatives may ask without the patient's explicit consent. In the latter instance one should temporise unless the patient clearly wants an answer. In the former, if temporising is not possible then the optimistic end of the prognostic scale should be used.

Table 3.1 *Important issues at the time of presenting the diagnosis*

- Where possible introduce the likely final diagnosis as a possibility before confirmation
- The news should be broken
  - by the most senior member of the team
  - with plenty of time
  - in a quiet and uninterrupted setting
- Answer questions that are put
  - honestly
  - positively
  - if the patient wants them answered
- Encourage the patient to articulate their fears
- Defer the discussion of other specifics until an early follow up appointment
- Point to all sources of support including charities, self-help groups, etc.
- Never extinguish hope. Be positive and encourage positivity

An early review appointment should be given for clarification of points already discussed and for the many questions the patient and family may by then have formulated. Liaison nurses, family care officers and other paramedical members of the multidisciplinary team (Table 3.2) can also be most valuable sources of support at this time. Now is a more appropriate time to talk about the specifics of supportive therapy and prognosis than at the initial consultation where diagnosis is announced.

The time of "telling" is a crucial one for the long-term management of progressive neuromuscular disorders. It is very hard to win many friends at this time, but very easy to create a poor relationship. This would have

Table 3.2 *Members of a neuromuscular multidisciplinary team*

Neurologist with experience in neuromuscular disease
Paediatrician/paediatric neurologist
Neurophysiologist
Muscle pathologist
Orthopaedic surgeon
Rehabilitation medicine specialist
Physiotherapist
Occupational therapist
Family care officer or specialist nurse
Plus input from educational psychology, occupational health, social work, etc.

long-term consequences for both patient and physician, and must be avoided.

Specific therapies

For only a few of the neuromuscular disorders are disease modifying therapies available (Table 3.3). Broadly speaking these consist of immunosuppressant agents for inflammatory and autoimmune disorders, symptomatic treatments of ion channel diseases (such as mexilitene in myotonia congenita or hyperkalaemic periodic paralysis or acetazolamide in hypokalaemic periodic paralysis), and manipulation of neuromuscular transmission for myasthenia or Lambert-Eaton myasthenic syndrome (LEMS). In this section we shall deal with the basic principles of the use of the above groups of drugs. Gene therapy for neuromuscular disease has been the subject of many trials but as yet

Table 3.3 *Neuromuscular diseases for which specific treatments exist*

- **Myopathies**
  Dermatomyositis
  Polymyositis and myositis in association with underlying connective tissue disease
  Myotonia congenita
  Sodium channel myotonias, including paramyotonia congenita
  Hyperkalaemic periodic paralysis
  Hypokalaemic periodic paralysis
  Endocrine and nutritional myopathies (treatment of underlying disorder)
  Carnitine deficiency
  (Duchenne muscular dystrophy – corticosteroids of slight benefit)
- **Neuromuscular junction disorders**
  Myasthenia gravis
  Congenital myasthenia
  Lambert-Eaton myasthenic syndrome
  Botulism
- **Peripheral nerve**
  Acute inflammatory neuropathies
  Chronic inflammatory demyelinating neuropathy
  Multifocal motor neuropathy with conduction block
  Vasculitic neuropathies
  Refsum's disease
  Toxic neuropathies
  Neuromyotonia

Table 3.4 *Drugs used in the treatment of myotonia and the channelopathies of muscle*

Channel involved →	Unknown	Chloride (CLC-1)	Calcium (CACNL1A3)	Sodium (SCN4A)	Sodium (SCN4A)	Sodium (SCN4A)
Drug ↓	Myotonic dystrophy	Myotonia congenita	Hypokalaemic periodic paralysis	Paramyotonia congenita	Hyperkalaemic periodic paralysis	Sodium channel myotonia
Phenytoin	☑ *	✓				
Procainamide	✓					
Quinine	✓					
Mexilitene		☑		☑ *		☑
Acetazolamide			✓		✓	✓
Thiazides			☒		☑	
Potassium			☑		☒	☒
Spironolactone			✓		☒	☒

☑	Drug of first choice
✓	Acceptable alternative
☒	Contraindicated
*	Where indicated

remains experimental and fraught with practical difficulties. It is not considered further in this book.

Treatment of muscle channelopathies and myotonia

The channelopathies of muscle (Chapter 6) are a heterogeneous group of disorders in which muscle overactivity in the form of myotonia is a frequent symptom. Myotonic dystrophy is also characterised by myotonia, although the origin of the myotonia in this condition does not appear to be a simple disorder of a single ion channel type. Drugs are available which provide effective relief from myotonia, and also others that may prevent the paralysis that occurs in the periodic paralyses, which are also due to ion channel dysfunction (Table 3.4). Before using any of these agents, however, it is important to ask the patient whether the myotonia is actually causing him or her any functional problems. When faced with a patient with myotonic dystrophy for example, it is very easy to focus on myotonia as "something we can help with" and then to treat it with a drug that may have an adverse effect upon cardiac function. Treat what the patient wants treating, and don't forget the whole patient!

Drugs available for myotonia

Drugs that reduce the excitability of the cell membrane, such as local anaesthetics and anti-arrhythmics are often effective in myotonia. They have their effect by reducing

sodium channel activity but are effective in channelopathies that affect not only sodium but also chloride channels (such as myotonia congenita). Phenytoin and procainamide have historically been the most widely used, but more recently the drug of first choice for non-dystrophic myotonias has become mexilitene. Before prescribing this drug, an ECG should be obtained and if there is any history of cardiac disease a cardiologist consulted. In many cases remarkable results are achieved with very small doses (100-200 mg daily), but some patients require 400-800 mg daily, in which case the slow release form of the drug is preferred. Absorption of the drug varies markedly between individuals and drug levels may be helpful in titrating the dose. Regular ECGs should be performed in all patients on mexilitene.

Only a minority of patients with myotonic dystrophy ask for drug treatment of their myotonia, and an even smaller number continue with treatment once it has been started. Given the high incidence of cardiac conduction disorders in this disease, phenytoin is a better drug of first choice than mexilitene or the other anti-arrhythmics. Care is necessary for women of child-bearing years to counsel about the teratogenic risks of phenytoin, and other side effects of treatment should be considered as when the drug is used in epilepsy.

Drugs for periodic paralysis

Acetazolamide may prevent attacks in both hyperkalaemic and hypokalaemic periodic paralysis. In hyperkalaemic periodic paralysis, a sodium channel disorder that is allelic with paramyotonia congenita, low dose thiazide diuretics are preferred, however, to the side effects of the acetazolamide. Both drugs are thought to work in this condition by reducing serum potassium.

In hypokalaemic periodic paralysis, due to a calcium channel disorder, either potassium supplements or potassium-sparing diuretics such as spironolactone are preferred for the same reason.

Treatment of neuromuscular junction disorders

Anticholinesterases

This group of drugs is used in the diagnosis and symptomatic control of myasthenia gravis (Chapter 12) and work by inhibiting the enzyme cholinesterase (ChE). This enzyme is present at the neuromuscular junction and breaks down acetylcholine (ACh) limiting the duration of action of ACh at the nicotinic receptors on the sarcolemma. By inhibiting the enzyme, levels of ACh in the neuromuscular clefts rise and are able to ameliorate the inhibition of neuromuscular transmission due to myasthenia. The drugs are sometimes used to provide symptomatic improvement in strength in some other disorders including motor neurone disease. One danger of this group of drugs is that if levels of ACh are too high in the neuromuscular junction a depolarization blockade of the ACh receptors may occur, itself worsening weakness.

The side effects of these drugs include unwanted parasympathetomimetic effects due to stimulation at muscarinic synapses. Diarrhoea, colic and excess salivation may occur and may require treatment with antimuscarinic agents such as atropine or propantheline. In general, pyridostigmine is better tolerated than neostigmine, although the latter has a more powerful effect and a quicker onset of action.

The short-acting ChE inhibitor, edrophonium, is used in diagnostic testing (the Tensilon test – Figure 3.1) since it has a duration of action of only five minutes or less. It may also be used to see if weakness is due to myasthenic blockade (which will improve after edrophonium) or cholinergic blockade (which will worsen). Edrophonium is a potent drug, however, and must be treated with respect. Full resuscitation facilities should be available when performing the test, and patients should be pre-treated with atropine unless there is a contra-indication. It is not a quick test to be performed in outpatients on a sleepy Friday afternoon.

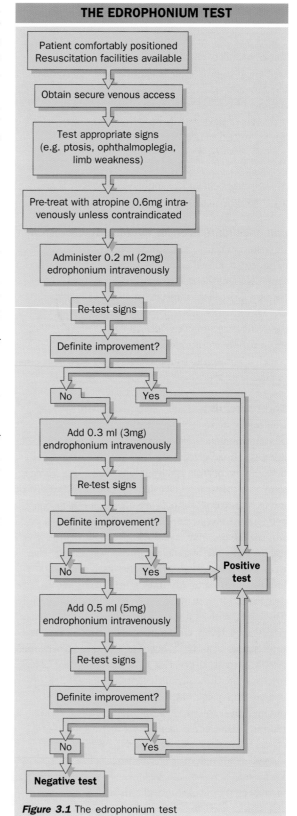

Figure 3.1 The edrophonium test

Presynaptic modulators of neuromuscular transmission

The agent 3,4 diaminopyridine (3,4-DAP) acts to block potassium channels and thus prolongs the presynaptic action potential. It thus enhances the influx of calcium and will increase quantal release of acetylcholine (ACh) at the neuromuscular junction. The main role of 3,4-DAP is in the treatment of Lambert-Eaton myasthenic syndrome, in which presynaptic calcium channel function is blocked by autoantibodies (Chapter 12). The drug is only available on a named-patient basis and its use should be supervised by suitably experienced clinicians.

Immunosuppression in neuromuscular disease

In neuromuscular disorders where the underlying pathology is either autoimmune or inflammatory then suppression of the immune response is rational first line therapy. Disorders that fall into this category include dermatomyositis, polymyositis, myasthenia gravis and the rarer autoimmune disorders of neuromuscular transmission. In this section we shall merely discuss the principles of immunosuppression, which are applicable to all disease types.

Corticosteroids

The corticosteroids comprise the mainstay of treatment of autoimmune and inflammatory neuromuscular diseases. Broadly speaking they may be used in short intravenous courses (usually at high dose) or as a longer-term oral treatment. The evidence base on which oral or intravenous corticosteroids are preferred is usually quite poor for an individual disease. High dose intravenous corticosteroids may rapidly curtail an autoimmune response and are in general associated with fewer long-term side effects than oral corticosteroids. In general, however, oral corticosteroids are preferred and may be used either on a daily or alternate day basis. Alternate day dosing with oral corticosteroids is generally associated with a lower incidence of side effects. In certain very active disorders, however, and in myopathies associated with connective tissue disease the "off day" may be quite difficult for the patient symptomatically.

The important side effects of corticosteroids are outlined in Table 3.5. Before commencing treatment the physician should explain the more important side effects to the patient and some of the measures that may be taken to reduce the incidence of these effects. Particular care should be taken in explaining the increased risk of infection, the risks of glucose intolerance and of premature osteoporosis. All patients on ≥ 30

Table 3.5 *Important adverse effects of corticosteroids*

Increased risk of infection (NB: risk of severe chickenpox in patients not hitherto exposed)
Glucose intolerance (may precipitate diabetic ketoacidosis)
Obesity
Cushing's syndrome
Salt and water retention
Potassium depletion
Hypertension
Osteoporosis
Aseptic necrosis of the hip
Mood elevation
Depression
Steroid psychosis
Gastric irritation/ulceration
Steroid myopathy
Adrenal suppression
Growth suppression in children

mg of prednisolone (or equivalent) on alternate days should receive primary prophylaxis with calcium and Vitamin D or a bisphosphonate. All patients on long-term (greater than nine months) treatment should have regular bone densitometry screening for osteoporosis. Newer corticosteroid preparations such as Deflazacort are relatively bone sparing and may be of assistance where corticosteroid therapy is required in a patient with osteoporosis, although they are significantly more expensive than generic prednisolone or dexamethasone.

Finally, patients must be reminded that they should not suddenly stop taking their medication and that, should they become unwell, they may need to increase the dose of medication during the period of illness. A "steroid card" should be given to all patients starting therapy.

Second-line immunosuppressants

The second-line drugs used for immunosuppression in autoimmune neuromuscular disease include azathioprine, methotrexate, ciclosporin and cyclophosphamide (Table 3.6). All are associated with an increased risk of infection as well as other specific side effects. The best tolerated of the drugs seems to be azathioprine and it is currently the most widely used. Where patients are unable to tolerate this drug one of the others is used. All require some degree of laboratory monitoring. In the case of azathioprine full blood counts and liver function tests are performed every week for the first two months, then every three months. There is also currently interest in the use of mycophenolate mofetil, also used

Table 3.6 *Immunosuppressant agents used in muscle disease*

Drug	Dose range	Side effects	Monitoring/precautions
Azathioprine	2-3 mg/kg/d	(Usually well tolerated) Nausea, dose-related bone marrow suppression, risk of infections, hypersensitivity reactions. Rarely pancreatitis or pneumonitis	FBC/LFTs weekly for 8 weeks then 3 monthly
Methotrexate	7.5-20 mg once per week (reduce if renal failure)	Dose-related bone marrow suppression. Anorexia, nausea, diarrhoea. Oral ulceration, stomatitis, gingivitis, pharyngitis. Risk of hepatotoxicity with prolonged use. Teratogenic.	FBC & LFTs monthly initially, then 3 monthly
Ciclosporin	2-6 mg/kg/d (reduce if renal failure)	Dose-dependent rises in urea & creatinine, occasional major renal toxicity. Headaches. Hypertrichosis, hypertension, gum hypertrophy, fatigue, hepatic dysfunction. May precipitate gout.	Drug levels (weekly, then monthly when stable; more often with concomitant drugs). FBC, urea, creatinine & electrolytes, LFTs twice before treatment then fortnightly for three months, then monthly. Blood pressure.
Cyclo-phosphamide	1-1.5 mg/kg daily or high-dose intravenous pulse therapy in severe vasculitic disease (reduce if renal failure)	Dose-related bone marrow suppression. Hair loss, anorexia, nausea & vomiting. Azoospermia (do not use in young males – bank sperm). Teratogenic. Haemorrhagic cystitis (esp. high dose iv therapy).	Regular monitoring of FBC and LFTs. Maintain good fluid input. In case of drug induced lymphopenia consider pneumocystis prophylaxis (two tablets of co-trimoxazole thrice weekly)

widely in the prevention of transplant rejection, as a possible treatment for autoimmune neuromuscular disease but the results of large clinical trials are awaited.

Other techniques for immune modulation

In severe autoimmune disorders where conventional treatments have failed, or when a more rapid treatment of the autoimmune process is required then more intensive anti-immune therapy is required. In general this will mean either plasma exchange or the infusion of pooled human intravenous immunoglobulin (IVIg). Although the two treatments are often thought of as interchangeable (and the evidence for either one being much better than the other in most diseases is lacking) they have different risks and in some disorders expert opinion favours one over the other. In UK hospital practice, both are roughly equivalent in cost.

Infusion of pooled human intravenous immunoglobulin

Intravenous immunoglobulin therapy is now widely used in other autoimmune neurological diseases such as acute and chronic demyelinating polyneuropathies, and multifocal motor neuropathy with conduction block. Its

action is thought to depend partly upon the presence of anti-idiotypic antibodies in the IVIg, which may bind to pathogenic autoantibodies. The efficacy in diseases in which there is no specific autoantibody, such as dermatomyositis is therefore of academic as well as clinical interest. It is relatively easy to administer, and does not require specialist facilities only available in larger regional centres. The standard dosage is either 0.4g/kg/day for five days or 1g/kg/day for two days. Many patients develop a 'flu-like illness and in some a more severe systemic allergic reaction may occur; this is usually associated with selective IgA deficiency, which should be screened for before treatment and constitutes a contraindication to therapy. There is a theoretical risk of the passage of blood borne viruses, although known viruses are screened out by the blood transfusion authorities. Patients should have liver function tests performed before and at regular intervals during and soon after treatment. If there is a rise in the transaminases, blood must be taken for hepatitis serology.

Plasma exchange

Plasma exchange is a more complicated measure. It is therefore reserved for severe disease, and for patients who can tolerate the demands made upon their cardiovascular system. The role of specific immunoadsorption columns, which may be more selective in the antibodies that they remove, is not yet clear.

Both IVIg and plasma exchange have a short-term effect which then wears off as new autoantibodies are produced. In chronic autoimmune disorders, repeated courses of treatment may be required, at considerable cost. They are therefore usually used as adjuncts to the immunosuppressant treatments outlined above.

Preventive and supportive therapies

Physiotherapy and gait analysis

Very few medical textbooks contain any detail about the role of physiotherapy in the treatment of neurological or other diseases. In muscle disease, however, physiotherapy is of such importance that a section on the principles of therapy is crucial.

Since muscle strength is often markedly reduced in muscle disease it is obvious that physical functioning will be impaired. One role of the physiotherapist is therefore to maintain or improve muscle strength. The selective involvement of different muscles and the abnormal postures adopted by patients in order to overcome functional disabilities may also lead to contractures and deformities. The physiotherapist has an important role in preventing these secondary complications. He or she will also work closely with orthopaedic surgeons and orthotists in seeking ways of keeping the patient ambulant. Respiratory physiotherapy is used to help prevent atelectasis and the consequent worsening of respiratory function. When the patient is no longer able to stand or walk independently the physiotherapist will advise on seating.

In order to provide the best service for the patient the physiotherapist should be part of a multidisciplinary team and be involved in the initial assessment of patients after diagnosis. The initial assessment allows not only the identification of immediate problems and the development of a rapport with the patient, but should also allow some prediction of future problems. This may help to avoid such future problems presenting as a crisis where decisions are made in haste (and sometimes repented of at leisure). In clinical terms the physiotherapist will make a broad assessment including measures of muscle strength, physical performance (including gait analysis) and of respiratory function. In some cases the use of sophisticated equipment to measure some of these parameters is appropriate. Such measures include

quantitative maximum voluntary isometric contraction (MVIC) measurement of muscle strength and complex gait analysis. Many experienced physiotherapists, however, prefer to use a more straightforward assessment which perhaps better measures the clinical ability and disability and a number of motor function scores for neuromuscular disease are available. In the research setting more rigorous measures are obviously required, and the physiotherapist will be the professional best placed to perform them.

The precise treatment undertaken at any stage of a muscle disease depends on the underlying pathology as well as the clinical state of the patient. In an inflammatory myopathy, for example, when there is an acute relapse with much inflammation, active exercise is likely to exacerbate muscle damage and the emphasis of physiotherapy is on passive exercises and splinting to maintain a full range of movement and prevent contractures (as soon as the most acute phase is over however, active exercise should be restarted). When the inflammation has come under control with drugs then the emphasis of therapy is on increasing muscle strength and regaining the function that has been lost.

In contrast, in childhood muscular dystrophy (particularly Duchenne dystrophy) early on in the disease the maintenance of strength by active exercise and the prevention of contractures by stretching are important to maintain the patient walking. As the disease progresses increasing emphasis on respiratory management and the maintenance of vital capacity with inspiratory and expiratory muscle training, breathing exercises and postural drainage is required. Close liaison with the orthotists and orthopaedic surgeon will help to time properly the use of major splinting and orthoses. In the latter stages of the disease advice on wheelchairs and seating, and more active respiratory measures dominate treatment. At all stages in the childhood dystrophies and myopathies the physiotherapist must be aware of normal motor and psychological development. This is important in order to enhance not only motor skills but also psychosocial skills, which are inextricably linked.

Other roles for the neuromuscular physiotherapist include the prevention of disuse atrophy in patients who come to surgery or who for other reasons spend periods of time immobile in bed. The physiotherapist can also be extremely helpful in the management of chronic low back pain in patients who have a hyperlordosis as a result of their proximal weakness. Manipulative physiotherapy and mobilisations can provide useful pain relief, as can some of the other techniques such as interferential ultrasound and transcutaneous electrical nerve stimulation (TENS). Finally, the advice of a physio-therapist can be valuable in planning treatments for specific functional disabilities such as scapular fixation in patients with FSH dystrophy.

This is only a brief review of the principles of physio-therapy and should help the clinician in understanding what their colleagues have to offer. A good physiother-apist is particularly important in the management of childhood muscle disease but is no less important in the management of adults.

Management of respiratory complications of neuromuscular disease

Although some neuromuscular disorders may present with acute, or acute-on-chronic respiratory failure in the majority of cases respiratory failure will occur in the context of a known neuromuscular disorder. An important part of the follow up of some neuromuscu-lar disorders is therefore in identifying patients at risk and preventing the need for crisis management. As with all aspects of neuromuscular disease it is best if potential scenarios are discussed with the patient before they occur. A hurried consultation in the early hours of the morning with a patient's family is seldom the best time to make decisions which the patient and physician may need to follow for months or years. A list of neuromuscular disorders which may present with respiratory failure and in which respiratory failure may occur as a chronic phenomenon is given in Table 3.7.

Table 3.7 *Neuromuscular diseases complicated by respiratory failure*

Muscle	Drugs/toxins
Dystrophies	Fish/shellfish/crab poisoning**
Dystrophinopathies (Duchenne & Becker*)	Snake/spider/scorpion venom**
Myotonic dystrophy**	Tick paralysis**
Limb-girdle dystrophies (esp. severe childhood	Botulism**
autosomal recessive MD = α-sarcoglycanopathy)	Antibiotics (e.g. streptomycin, neomycin, Clindamycin,
Facioscapulohumeral dystrophy*	polymixin B)**
Scapuloperoneal MD	**Peripheral nerve**
Congenital myopathies	Inflammatory neuropathies
X-linked myotubular myopathy**	Acute inflammatory demyelinating polyneuropathy**
Nemaline myopathy**	Acute motor axonal neuropathy**
Rigid spine syndrome**	Chronic inflammatory demyelinating polyneuropathy
Metabolic myopathies	Vasculitic neuropathies
Acid maltase deficiency**	Metabolic neuropathies
Primary carnitine deficiency**	Acute intermittent porphyria
Mitochondrial disease (usually due to CNS disease)	Hereditary tyrosinaemia
Secondary to endocrine / electrolyte disturbances	Infections
Hypokalaemia**	Diphtheria
Hypophosphataemia**	Drugs/toxins
Barium intoxication**	Lead**
Hyperthyroidism (thyroid storm)**	Thallium**
Inflammatory myopathies	Arsenic**
Dermatomyositis*	Gold**
Polymyositis*	Lithium**
Neuromuscular junction	Organophosphates**
Myasthenia gravis**	Anterior horn cell
Lambert–Eaton mtasthetic syndrome (LEMS)**	Amyotrophic lateral sclerosis**
Congenital myasthenia**	Spinal muscular atrophy (esp. type I)**
	Late poliomyelitis

*Uncommon causes of respiratory failure; ** May present de novo with acute respiratory failure*

Ventilatory failure in neuromuscular disease is rather more complicated than may be initially apparent. The characteristic ventilatory fault in neuromuscular disease is a restrictive defect with a fall in vital capacity. Total lung volume and functional residual capacity are reduced while the residual volume is normal. Peak expiratory flow rates, forced expiratory volumes and similar measures are frequently preserved, however, so that simple measurements of peak flow are inadequate. As vital capacity reduces, areas of microatelectasis occur causing reduced lung compliance, an increase in the physiological dead space and a ventilation-perfusion mismatch. Intercostal muscle weakness and secondary stiffness of chest wall ligaments, tendons and joints further reduce chest wall compliance. If scoliosis occurs this will further reduce lung capacities. Another early change may be a reduced ability to cough, both due to reduced expiratory pressures, and impaired glottic function. Secretions may be retained further increasing the work of breathing and worsening the situation.

When the patient is asleep, he or she may be particularly vulnerable to the above effects, and respiratory insufficiency often begins as a sleep related phenomenon. Upper airway obstruction may occur due to weak pharyngeal musculature. During REM sleep the chemotaxic drive is reduced and when combined with a reduced background CNS ventilatory drive, as occurs in some neuromuscular diseases, episodes of hypoxaemia and hypercapnia may develop. At first these episodes are short-lived but as the diseases progress they become longer, disrupting normal sleep and leading to chronic daytime hypoxaemia and hypercapnia.

A further complication that may occur during sleep is that the vital capacity is reduced in most neuromuscular diseases when the patient is supine. This is because of diaphragmatic weakness, which allows the abdominal contents to push the diaphragm upward into the thoracic cavity, as well as reducing the inspiratory force arising from the diaphragm. Chronic constipation, gastric dilatation or obesity will worsen the situation.

As areas of microatelectasis and ventilation-perfusion mismatch increase, there is hypoxic vasoconstriction of pulmonary vessels and an increasing load on the right heart so that cor pulmonale may develop. Hypoxia and hypercapnia further impair function of both skeletal and cardiac muscle, worsening the cycle of events already described above and also putting the patient at risk of potentially fatal arrhythmias. At this stage oxygen therapy may further reduce respiratory drive, and paradoxically prolong apnoeas or hypopnoeas, and must therefore be avoided.

Table 3.8 *Symptoms suggesting ventilatory insufficiency*

Dyspnoea
Sleep disturbance
Nightmares
Anxiety
Nausea
Vomiting
Headaches
Hypersomnolence
Poor concentration
Poor memory
Drooling

All may occur first in the context of intercurrent respiratory infections

Table 3.9 *Signs of ventilatory insufficiency*

EARLY
Tachypnoea
Irregular or shallow breathing
Use of accessory muscles
Abdominal paradox during respiration
Difficulty speaking in long sentences
Poor swallowing

LATER
Drooling
Nasal speech
Nasal regurgitation of fluids
Dysphagia
Hypertension
Signs of right heart failure (oedema, ↑ JVP, tricuspid regurgitation)
Mental slowing
Papilloedema

These changes are summarised in Figure 3.2 and from the account given above of this complex downward spiral of respiratory function, it is clear that early rather than late identification of ventilatory failure action is required for optimal care. Indeed, early intervention may delay ventilator-dependency, rather than merely bringing forward decisions about invasive ventilation. Thus any clinician caring for chronic neuromuscular disease must be aware of the symptoms and signs which suggest early ventilatory insufficiency, and what action may then be taken.

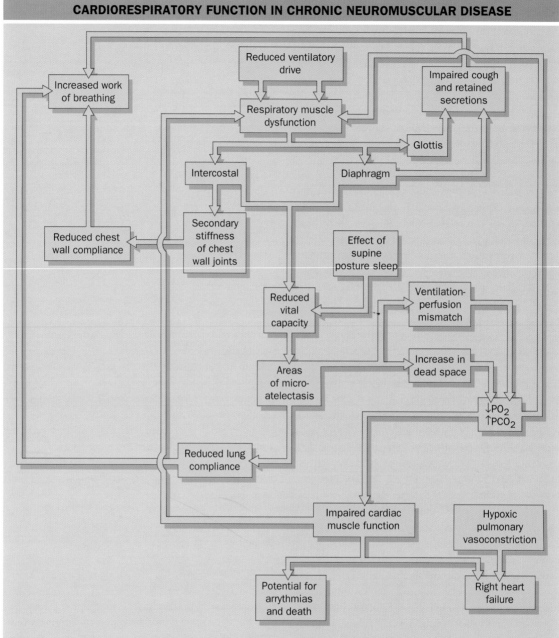

CARDIORESPIRATORY FUNCTION IN CHRONIC NEUROMUSCULAR DISEASE

Figure 3.2 Cardiorespiratory function in chronic neuromuscular disease. The interconnected changes that lead to chronic respiratory failure and its consequences. Changes that are exacerbated in sleep are shown by red arrows.

Assessment of ventilatory function

At follow up the patient and their carers should be questioned closely for symptoms suggesting ventilatory insufficiency (Table 3.8) taking care to remember that such symptoms may occur first during intercurrent respiratory infections. Signs of respiratory insufficiency (Table 3.9) should also be closely sought.

The simplest and best assessment that should be undertaken in the clinic at least annually (and more often if the clinical context suggests rapid deterioration) is recording of the vital capacity (VC) and relating it to the normal values for the patients age, height and weight. Broadly speaking patients start to develop problems when the VC falls to 30% of predicted. At this stage (or earlier, at about 40% of predicted) it is therefore important that the patient and their family are warned of the risks of both chronic respiratory failure and the risks of an acute deterioration in the face of intercurrent illness (see below).

Other useful and relatively simple measures are the peak cough expiratory flow and the inspiratory sniff pressures. These can be measured using relatively cheap hand-held meters and are valuable in detecting patients at risk of respiratory complications and the measurements can help in planning what kind of ventilatory support is likely to be successful. Finally more comprehensive pulmonary function testing, including measurement of static pressures and compliance loops may be indicated particularly if there are respiratory symptoms, but clearly cannot be performed in the outpatient clinic.

Management of chronic ventilatory insufficiency
Once the VC has fallen to 40-50% of predicted, the patient should start respiratory exercises (except in myasthenia where fatigue may worsen respiratory function). The patient and their carer should be taught the techniques of assisted coughing to help to clear secretions, and later in the disease those of postural drainage. A chest x-ray (CXR) and electrocardiogram (ECG) should also be obtained to look for other pulmonary pathology and evidence of right heart strain or failure. Immunisations against influenza and pneumococcal infections should be given.

In centres with an extremely active approach to respiratory failure, arterial blood gases are obtained and if abnormal daytime and night time ventilation discussed and instituted. If they are normal, overnight oximetry and capnography are performed and if abnormal then trials of nocturnal ventilation given.

In all cases and in all centres, the decisions about when and whether to institute mechanical ventilation of any kind are complex, and require full and open discussion with the patient and their family. The social situation (including the availability of carers and in some societies the financial resources), the nature and tempo of the disease and the wishes of the patient all need to be taken into account. Usually the patient will be only too aware of the likelihood that they will have breathing problems eventually and will often value the opportunity to express their fears and to get some realistic facts about timescale and possible treatments.

It is equally important for the patient to know that they can always stop using the ventilator and that that decision will remain theirs. This basic principle needs to be made explicit from the outset so that, if the patient decides that they no longer wish to live a life that involves mechanical support, they can easily raise the subject of discontinuation.

Types of ventilation
A detailed discussion of ventilators is outside the scope of this book, but an idea of the types of ventilation available is important, as are a few of the principles governing their use.

Although fixed in the minds of the public following their widespread use in the aftermath of the great polio epidemics, whole body ventilators ("iron lungs" and their successors) are now only rarely used in clinical practice. They work either by creating sub-atmospheric pressure around the thorax and abdomen to directly cause airflow, or on the abdomen alone to move the abdominal contents and secondarily the diaphragm (e.g. "rocking beds"). Most are clumsy and cumbersome and they may worsen the closure of the hypopharynx, which causes obstructive apnoea.

The aim of most ventilatory support is to provide home based mechanically assisted ventilation. For best results, patients with a VC about 30% of predicted should be considered for nocturnal support. In a few cases, where obstructive apnoeas are the major problem continuous positive airway pressure (CPAP) will suffice. More commonly intermittent positive pressure ventilation (IPPV) is needed. Nocturnal IPPV is given wherever possible via a nasal mask (so called "Nippy" – NIPPV), but if there is weakness of lip seal due to orofacial weakness a mask covering both lips and mouth is sometimes required. Simple mouthpieces may be used for intermittent daytime support – to give a few deep insufflations and improve oxygen saturation or give sufficient force for a cough. As the VC falls still further the patient is likely to require increasing periods of time on the ventilator and by the time it falls to 10-15% of predicted most require 24-hour support.

In a proportion of patients IPPV can only be given via a tracheostomy. This is usually the case when there is severe bulbar muscle dysfunction, either causing problems with leakage from nose or mouth during non-invasive ventilation or with major aspiration of secretions. Tracheostomies require an even higher level of care than non-invasive IPPV but can still provide a level of independence and with appropriate tubes speech is still possible.

Acute neuromuscular respiratory failure

In the context of known neuromuscular disease, acute respiratory failure is usually precipitated by some inter-current process such as infection, aspiration or heart failure. Also a variety of drugs may precipitate acute respiratory failure especially in myasthenia gravis (Table 3.10) but also rarely in other disorders. For example, calcium channel blockers have been reported to worsen respiratory failure in Duchenne muscular dystrophy and β-receptor blockers may generally impair muscle function. Benzodiazepines may reduce central respiratory drive and precipitate respiratory failure in a patient with neuromuscular disease. Electrolyte imbalance, particularly hypokalaemia or hypophosphataemia may also trigger respiratory failure.

It is important to remember, however, that the patient may develop respiratory failure for reasons entirely unconnected with their neuromuscular disease. Chronic obstructive lung disease, heart failure and infection may be solely responsible, particularly in those neuromuscular diseases where ventilatory insufficiency is very rare, such as facioscapulohumeral muscular dystrophy and some of the distal myopathies.

A number of the neuromuscular disorders may present for the first time with respiratory failure, either because other muscles are relatively unaffected or because the patient has not sought help for their other symptoms. Thus the neurologist may be asked to assess patients with acute respiratory failure in whom there is no existing diagnosis.

Patients who are dyspnoeic or obtunded clearly need emergency endotracheal intubation. In less acute settings, frequent measurement of vital capacity is mandatory. Where the VC is less than 30ml/kg there is impaired clearance of secretions, and at less than 10 ml/kg the patient is in frank ventilatory failure and must be intubated.

In cases where mechanical ventilation is likely to be prolonged, a tracheostomy should be performed early to minimise vocal cord and tracheal damage – preferably using a technique likely to produce a good long-term result such as a percutaneous Seldinger technique. The tracheostomy also allows much less sedation to be used and allows access to the trachea for suction and chest physiotherapy. Usually positive end expiratory pressure (PEEP) is used together with physiotherapy to try to minimise atelectasis. Other basic principles of intensive

Table 3.10 *Drugs and therapeutic agents that may worsen or precipitate respiratory failure in myasthenia gravis (this list is not exhaustive)*

Anaesthetic agents
- Suxamethonium
- D-tubocurarine and similar agents
- Gallamine
- Ether

Antibiotics
- Clindamycin
- Colistin
- Gentamicin
- Neomycin
- Streptomycin
- Tetracyclines

Anticonvulsants
- Phenytoin

Cardiac drugs
- Diltiazem
- Beta blockers
- Calcium channel blockers
- Lignocaine
- Quinidine
- Procainamide

Hormonal preparations
- ACTH
- Corticosteroids
- Oral contraceptives
- Thyroxine

Psychotropic agents
- Benzodiazepines
- Chlorpromazine and related drugs
- Lithium

Rheumatological drugs (immunosuppressants)
- Chloroquine
- Penicillamine

Miscellaneous
- Quinine
- Iodinated intravenous contrast agents
- Ringer's lactate

care such as prevention of infection, nutrition and attention to pressure areas are obviously also important.

Once on a ventilator rapid diagnosis of the underlying disease, where there is no pre-existing neuromuscular diagnosis, or of the precipitating factor where a reasonable neuromuscular diagnosis does exist, is required. Treatment of the precipitating cause (and of the underlying disease, where possible) is then instituted.

Cardiac management

Many of the diseases of skeletal muscle may also affect cardiac muscle, despite its different structure and function. In a number of these diseases the involvement of cardiac muscle is out of proportion to any involvement of skeletal muscle and may precede any neuromuscular manifestations at all. Moreover many of the cardiac complications are more amenable to treatment than those of skeletal muscle and their recognition may markedly improve both quality and quantity of life.

All patients with a potential neuromuscular diagnosis should therefore undergo some form of elementary cardiac assessment. This should include direct questioning about cardiac symptoms such as palpitations, syncope, pre-syncope, dyspnoea and oedema. A proper examination of the cardiovascular system should be performed and an electrocardiogram (ECG) taken. In cases where there are symptoms to suggest cardiac disease an echocardiogram, chest radiograph and other investigations (e.g. Holter monitoring or radionuclide scanning) are also required. As a simple rule, if in doubt about a patient's diagnosis, err on the side of caution and perform an ECG and examine the heart.

The specific details of how individual diseases may affect the heart are given in the individual disease descriptions, but in this chapter we shall briefly cover the principles of how cardiac muscle is affected and the clinical results. Table 3.11 shows the common pattern of cardiac involvement in the diseases as an overview.

Conducting system disease

Involvement of the conducting system itself usually causes progressive heart block. This is the commonest pattern seen, for example, in myotonic dystrophy where patients under continuing follow-up show increasing prolongation of the PR interval of the ECG. Histologically there is fibrosis and some fatty replacement which is very focused on the conducting system. Timely implantation of a pacemaker can be lifesaving in this condition, as it may also in Emery-Dreifuss muscular dystrophy. In the latter condition sudden cardiac death may occur in up to 50% of untreated patients.

Tachyarrhythmias

As well as causing Stokes-Adams attacks and other forms of syncope by causing bradyarrhythmias, more diffuse involvement of cardiac muscle in the myopathies may result in atrial or ventricular tachyarrhythmias, which present as fainting or palpitations. Sometimes the myocardial involvement is severe enough to result in marked signs of a dilated (or more rarely hypertrophic) cardiomyopathy. An example is the cardiomyopathy of Duchenne muscular dystrophy. In other diseases a more patchy pattern of myocardial involvement predisposes to the production of local re-entrant electrical circuits, but is not sufficient to significantly interfere with pump function. Again, an example of such a disease is myotonic dystrophy.

Dilated cardiomyopathy

Where involvement of cardiac muscle is sufficiently severe, the pumping function of the heart is directly impaired and signs of heart failure will follow. The myocardium may be directly involved in the disease, as in the dystrophinopathies where lack of dystrophin is associated with a dilated cardiomyopathy late on in the disease. Abnormalities on ECG and echocardiography are present in over half of patients with dystrophinopathy but do not always correlate well with clinical state. Indeed, a clinically significant proportion of asymptomatic female carriers are reported to have ECG abnormalities but there is no evidence as yet that they are at increased risk of cardiac symptoms.

Table 3.11 *Patterns of cardiac involvement in some common myopathies*

Disease	Bradyarrhythmias	Tachyarrhythmias	Cardiomyopathy	Sudden death
Duchenne	±	Atrial +	Dilated, late +	+
		ventricular + (later)	hypertrophic, early ±	
Becker	+	+	30%	+
Emery-Dreifuss	Sinus bradycardia ++	Atrial ++	+	50%
	AV block (later) +++			
Myotonic dystrophy	++	+	±	+
Kearns-Sayre syndrome	++	–	Dilated, late	+
Primary Inflammatory myopathies	±	–	±	–

Other ways in which the myocardium may be compromised in muscle diseases include direct invasion by inflammatory cells in inflammatory myopathies, metabolic dysfunction in some mitochondrial disorders, storage of abnormal glycogen in some glycogenoses and by electrolyte disturbances in the periodic paralyses.

Secondary orthopaedic problems

For many years the long-term follow-up and management of neuromuscular diseases was largely the province of orthopaedic surgeons. In recent years there has been a marked shift away from surgical treatment in patients with chronic neuromuscular diseases, but the judicious use of orthotics and orthopaedic surgical procedures may still be of functional benefit to the patient. A full review of orthopaedic and orthotic management would be inappropriate in a book of this type, but we shall briefly discuss some general principles.

Much of the orthopaedic expertise in dealing with deformities resulting from neuromuscular disease arose from the experience in dealing with survivors of the great poliomyelitis epidemics. In the majority of the diseases described in this book, however, there is a crucial difference which is that the diseases themselves are continually progressing and the functional effects on the patients changing. Moreover, in the childhood diseases the patients are themselves continually changing due to growth. It follows that any surgical or orthotic solution must be robust enough to deal with what will happen in the future as well as current functional disability. Indeed it is important that there is a sound functional reason for intervention, since ill-considered attempts to produce a cosmetic improvement may often lead to functional worsening of disability. Surgical treatment of pes cavus and hammer toes in neuromuscular patients can lead to functional deterioration, as may over aggressive use of tendon release or transfer operations in mild foot drop when the use of physiotherapy and orthotics might be a better option. Finally the damage that a period of enforced bed rest after surgery can cause to a patient with an active muscle disease cannot be overemphasised.

There clearly is a role for the orthopaedic surgeon as part of the multidisciplinary neuromuscular team, however. The best efforts of physiotherapists and orthotists will eventually be unable to deal with many cases of equinovarus deformity in late Duchenne dystrophy, for example. In this instance well-timed Achilles tenotomies with the fitting of knee-ankle-foot orthoses or post-operative splinting may prolong ambulation. Also in Duchenne dystrophy and other progressive neuromuscu-

lar disorders, the development of scoliosis markedly impairs not only ambulation, but also respiratory function. The use of thoracolumbar spinal orthoses or segmental spinal instrumentation (e.g. with Harrington's rods) can be extremely effective in correcting deformity in this instance and producing a functional gain.

The basic principles governing the use of orthotic devices are similar to those described above for surgical intervention. The devices have the advantage that they can be removed and are therefore less likely to cause permanent problems if they are not correct. Patients should not, however, lose any functional adaptation that they had made. It is important that the devices are individually made and fitted, and that the patient can come back for further adaptations if they are not happy. It is very easy to forget that a small area of redness or a secondary callosity can be extremely uncomfortable and may result in the patient simply not wearing the orthosis. Ankle foot orthoses for foot drop are particularly prone to be poorly fitted and for the patients to therefore consign them to the back of a cupboard. As a young patient grows it is important for the orthosis to be frequently reviewed both for comfort and to ensure that it is still performing the task required of it.

In summary, orthopaedic intervention in neuromuscular disease is not a "last resort", but should only be performed after a careful multidisciplinary assessment. Ideally the neuromuscular team should contain both a dedicated orthotist and also someone with expertise in biomechanics and/or gait analysis who can advise on the likely benefits and pitfalls of any planned procedures.

Anaesthesia and neuromuscular disease

The involvement of respiratory and cardiac muscle in many myopathies makes the patients at some significant risk from anaesthesia. To this must be added the risk of malignant hyperpyrexia, which exists in some conditions, as well as idiosyncrasies in the reactions to other drugs (particularly neuromuscular blocking drugs) which exist in some myopathies. Finally smooth muscle dysfunction, where present, may cause delayed gastric emptying and increase the risk of aspiration.

It follows that the preoperative assessment of respiratory function and cardiac function must be meticulous, as should assessment of bulbar function (to assess cough strength and the risks of aspiration). Respiratory function testing and arterial blood gas analysis should be performed in any patient at risk of respiratory complications. Chest physiotherapy pre-operatively is also important.

The anaesthetic procedure will need to take into account not only the potential post-operative complications (see below) but also direct risks of anaesthetic agents in this group of patients. The most well known is the risk of malignant hyperpyrexia (MH), where muscle rigidity, rapid rise in body temperature and metabolic acidosis follow use of some drugs including anaesthetic agents. This is discussed in more detail in Chapter 6, but in a patient who may have a myopathy that is either as yet undiagnosed or is "undiagnosable" then the safe cause of action is to assume that the patient IS at risk of MH and the anaesthetic regime tailored with this in mind. The other major anaesthetic problem to consider is the effect of neuromuscular blocking drugs. Obviously in diseases of the neuromuscular junction there is a risk of incomplete reversal of neuromuscular blockade. In other diseases non-depolarizing relaxants may also be associated with prolonged duration of action and careful peri- and postoperative monitoring is essential. The response to depolarizing agents may be more dramatic, however. In myotonic dystrophy (and sometimes other myotonias) there may be a rapid and severe increase in muscle tone. In this and some other conditions rhabdomyolysis, malignant hyperpyrexia and cardiac arrest have been reported also. Suxamethonium should therefore be avoided in patients with muscle disease wherever possible.

Post operatively, the central effects of anaesthetic agents, sedatives and analgesics may combine to depress respiratory drive and in the vulnerable patient with a reduced respiratory reserve this may lead to problems weaning from the ventilator and even the development of acute Type II respiratory failure after what seems to be initially successful anaesthetic reversal/recovery. Medical and nursing staff need to be alert to these possibilities and to take such precautions (including regular measurement of vital capacity, chest physiotherapy and incentive spirometry) as are necessary to prevent problems or to detect them early.

The basic principles of anaesthetic management in muscle disease are given in Table 3.12.

Genetic counselling, support and screening

Many of the diseases described in this book are inherited and all of these inherited diseases are, at present, incurable. This poses a great burden both physical and psychological not only for patients but also for their families. Accurate information not only about the diagnosis but also about the risks of other family members being affected is important, as is the question

Table 3.12 Principles of anaesthetic management in neuromuscular diseases

Preoperative assessment
Is diagnosis clear and accurate?
Is there a risk of MH?
Is there evidence of neuromuscular block?
Cough, swallowing
Bedside assessment of thoracic and abdominal wall motion
Respiratory function tests
Blood gases
Cardiac status: ECG ± echocardiography

Perioperative care
Avoid suxamethonium
Monitoring of temperature, and for signs of MH
Routine cardiac monitoring
Monitor neuromuscular blockade

Postoperative care
Ensure adequate reversal of anaesthesia and neuromuscular blockade
Monitoring of respiratory function using vital capacity
Chest physiotherapy ± incentive spirometry
Avoid prolonged bed rest

of prenatal or presymptomatic diagnosis. This is the role of genetic counselling.

Genetic counselling is often more about families than just individuals, although the needs of each individual within the family must also be addressed. Before counselling of any member can begin the diagnosis in the "index" case must be confirmed, and it is often not that case who is referred for counselling. Thus all the available diagnostic information from the index case must be reviewed, and sometimes it is necessary to see that the index case patient in person where it is practical to do so (and if the index case patient agrees).

A clear idea of the mode of inheritance of the condition in question is obviously essential. A family tree (pedigree) must be drawn up covering as many generations as possible. This time consuming task can often be performed by special trained genetic nurses or counsellors, and these individuals can also explain much about the principles of genetic counselling and to answer questions and allay fears in the patient.

The patient who is being counselled will usually have one of three reasons for seeking counselling. The first is to see if they themselves carry a disease that may cause problems with their own health now or in the future. Even if the disease has no prospect of a "cure", it may be important to identify patients who carry the disease at a presymptomatic stage to avoid other serious risks to themselves. Examples would include screening of relatives of patients with central core disease because of the risk of malignant hyperpyrexia and the early diagnosis of myotonic dystrophy where cardiac conduction defects may occur in patients with minimal limb symptoms.

The second reason for seeking counselling is to assess the risk to your own living relatives including children. This may be because of the "presymptomatic complications" outlined above or because of the risk of these living relatives then having an affected child themselves. An example would be where a middle-aged man discovered that his older sister had just been diagnosed with myotonic dystrophy. Rather than his two daughters being tested themselves, if he were tested and found to be negative for the appropriate expansion mutation, then his daughters would be at no significant risk of being gene carriers. In general geneticists try to avoid performing tests on an individual where the result would then mean that another person (usually the parent) would have an "obligate" diagnosis made where they did not want this information or had not been counselled before testing. In the example above if one of the daughters had been tested and found to be positive, the father would then almost certainly be a carrier (assuming paternity etc). This might be information which he was not prepared for, or did not want. Therefore the ideal approach is for the genetics team to discuss testing with the father as well, although if he would not be tested and the daughter wanted an answer (e.g. for consideration of prenatal diagnosis) then she would be tested. This, of course comprises the third reason for seeking genetic advice – to identify the risks to ones future offspring and whether prenatal genetic testing is available or indeed appropriate.

It follows from the discussion above that genetic counselling and testing must be performed in a careful and thoughtful way, taking into account the wishes of many family members. It is important to provide as much information as possible to the patient and to explain not only the reasons why the patient should be tested, but also reasons why they might not wish to be tested. Not only the psychological effect upon the individual of a positive diagnosis, but more mundane but important aspects such as the future ability to get insurance cover need to be addressed. A blood test without counselling is not acceptable.

Whoever does the genetic counselling must be well experienced and aware of all of these considerations. Frequently a specialist in genetics is in the best position to do this, but there are occasions where the specialist involved has sufficient experience to undertake at least some of the counselling themselves. Many physicians who run muscle disease services will see much inherited disease and can undertake genetic counselling as part of their integrated service.

Support organisations

The muscle diseases, like many other neurological diseases, tend to be progressive lifelong disorders, which make a profound physical and mental impact on the patient and their carers. Support organisations and charities are invaluable sources of information and frequently also of practical help, and should be used as much as possible. Newly diagnosed patients should be given a contact address or telephone number for the local charity and encouraged to contact them. When dealing with an incurable disease, other than a good group of carers and strength of character, one important weapon is information about your disease. If we are unable to cure the disease it is incumbent upon us as physicians to provide the patients with the weapons they need to help themselves.

Selected further reading

Dalakas MC. Current treatment of the inflammatory myopathies. *Curr Opin Rheum* 1994; 6: 595–601.

Dalakas MC. Intravenous immunoglobulin therapy for neurological diseases. *Ann Intern Med* 1997; 126: 721–730.

[Editorial]. The heart in myotonic dystrophy. *Lancet* 1992; 339: 528–529.

Edwards RHT, Griggs RC. Medical and psychological management of neuromuscular disease. In: Walton J, Karpati G, Hilton-Jones D (eds). *Disorders of Voluntary Muscle* 6th edn. Cambridge: Cambridge University Press, 1994.

Engel AG, Franzini-Armstrong C (eds). *Myology*, 2nd edn, New York: McGraw-Hill, 1994.

Hirsch NP, Russell SH. Anesthesia and primary muscle disease. In: Lane RJM (ed). *Handbook of Muscle Disease.* New York: Marcel Dekker, 1996: 629–638.

Hughes RAC, Bihari D. Acute neuromuscular respiratory paralysis. *J Neurol Neurosurg Psychiatry* 1993; 56: 334–343.

Hyde S. Physical therapy of muscle diseases. In: Lane RJM (ed). *Handbook of Muscle* Disease. New York: Marcel Dekker, 1996.

Karpati G, Hilton-Jones D, Griggs R (eds). *Disorders of Voluntary Muscle* 7th edn. Cambridge: Cambridge University Press, 2001.

Lane RJM (ed). *Handbook of Muscle Disease.* New York: Marcel Dekker, 1996.

Quinlivan RM, Dubowitz V. Cardiac transplantation in Becker muscular dystrophy. *Neuromusc Dis* 1992; 2: 165–167.

Tawil R, McDermott MP, Brown R, Jr. et al. Randomized trials of dichlorphenamide in the periodic paralyses. Working Group on Periodic Paralysis. *Ann Neurol* 2000; 47: 46–53.

THE MYOPATHIES

chapter 4

The muscular dystrophies

To many lay people, muscular dystrophy is synonymous with Duchenne muscular dystrophy. As a result there are many misunderstandings and misconceptions, often compounded by a poor understanding of the conditions by healthcare professionals. It is very common, for example, to find families with an autosomal dominant dystrophy such as myotonic dystrophy that have been told that females cannot be affected by the condition. It follows that management is often less than optimum.

The term "muscular dystrophy" properly refers to an inherited, progressive disorder of muscle characterised by destruction of muscle and replacement by fatty and fibrous tissue. There are many different types, many of which are extremely rare. Since the 1950s there have been great advances in the clinical and molecular genetic classification of this group of disorders. It has to be said, however, that the advances made in accurate diagnosis are to some extent offset by the proliferation of confusing terms to describe the diseases and the gene products responsible for them.

In this chapter we shall present an overview of the dystrophies together with a more detailed account of the commoner dystrophies, and to try to provide the reader with a framework to understand these diseases.

Clinical diagnosis of muscular dystrophy

It should be no surprise to the reader that optimum clinical diagnosis of the dystrophies starts with a careful history and examination (Chapter 1). Particular care should be taken in the history to draw out any symptoms of disease that may have been present long before the patient became fully aware that he or she had any problem with the muscles. Thus it is important when taking the history from the mother of a child with a possible muscle problem to include the child's motor milestones, including head control, sitting and crawling and also whether foetal movements were normal and whether there was polyhydramnios. In an older patient

it is important to discover if they were able to take part in normal sports at school and if there was any history of painful cramps or exhaustion. Sometimes the patient may have been a very reluctant sportsman, or may have always been the last person to be chosen for football or hockey teams because they were too slow and this may be relevant and prompt closer questioning. Direct questioning about episodes of myoglobinuria is necessary. It is important to take a thorough family history, including any family members who might have been said to have walked strangely or to have had "arthritis". Also one should ask sensitively about any children who died young or were still born and to question tactfully about consanguinity.

On examination it is important to accurately chart the distribution of both wasting and weakness. The gait should be carefully assessed. In cases of diagnostic doubt it is often helpful to also examine other family members who may have sub-clinical signs of disease.

The dystrophinopathies

The best-known forms of muscular dystrophy are Duchenne and the milder Becker muscular dystrophies. Both are X-linked recessive disorders and the discovery of the gene product that is defective in the disorders, dystrophin, has confirmed that they are allelic disorders. A number of other muscle disorders, including syndromes of painful muscle cramps with or without episodes of myoglobinuria, have also been associated with mutations within the dystrophin gene thus broadening the spectrum of disorders linked to the gene. They are thus collectively known as the dystrophinopathies (Table 4.1).

Duchenne and Becker muscular dystrophies
Duchenne muscular dystrophy (DMD) is the commonest childhood muscular dystrophy with an incidence of about 1 in 3,500 live male births and a total male prevalence of about $50\text{-}70 \times 10^{6}$. Becker muscular dystrophy

Table 4.1 *The human dystrophinopathies*

Duchenne muscular dystrophy (DMD)

(Intermediate cases)

Becker muscular dystrophy (BMD)

Manifesting female carriers of DMD or BMD

Dystrophinopathy with myalgia and cramps

Isolated quadriceps myopathy

Isolated cardiomyopathies

Isolated hyperCKaemia

Table 4.2 *Diagnostic criteria for Duchenne and Becker muscular dystrophy*

Age of loss of anmulation	Diagnostic group
<13 years	Duchenne
13–16 years	Intermediate-type
>16 years	Becker

All require absence of DMD or reduced abundance (BMD) of dystrophin on immunostaining or immunoblotting.

(BMD) was thought to be far rarer, but it is clear that it is more common than thought with an incidence of about 1 in 18,000 live male births and a prevalence of 23.8×10^{-6}. There is a spectrum of severity between the two conditions, and to divide them requires clear diagnostic criteria (Table 4.2). There are some molecular genetic differences between the two ends of the spectrum but in general the diseases do form a spectrum rather than being discrete genetic diseases.

Genetics and pathophysiology

The dystrophinopathies are inherited in an X-linked recessive fashion, so that it is males who show the typical clinical picture. Females are not usually affected clinically but frequently show minor abnormalities on investigation such as a raised CK or mild abnormalities on routine EMG or biopsy. Some of these carriers show a mild and non-progressive clinical myopathy. A far smaller number may present as manifesting carriers. These patients may show a severe and progressive disorder in some cases indistinguishable from the disease seen in males. The most likely explanation is that these patients show a skewed pattern of the inactivation of the X-chromosome so that a higher than expected proportion of those chromosomes with a defective dystrophin gene remains active and producing mutant protein (Figure 4.1).

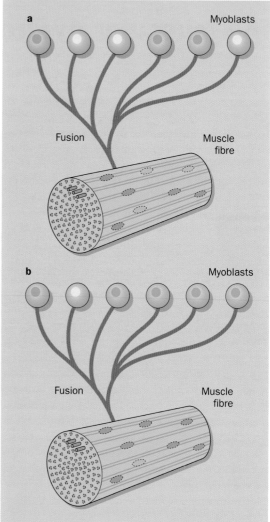

X-INACTIVATION AND SKEWED X-INACTIVATION

Figure 4.1 X-inactivation and skewed X-inactivation. (a) With random inactivation of the X chromosome, the myoblasts fuse to form a muscle fibre with sufficient nuclei producing dystrophin for near normal sarcolemmal dystrophin levels. (b) With a skewed pattern of inactivation, the majority of nuclei cannot produce dystrophin leading to dystrophin deficiency in the mature muscle fibre.

Approximately one in three cases of DMD are born into families previously known to be affected by the disease, but in two-thirds there is no family history (Figure 4.2). In the latter group, investigation reveals that the mother herself is a previously undiagnosed carrier

ORIGIN OF DMD GENES AND THE GENETIC CONSEQUENCES

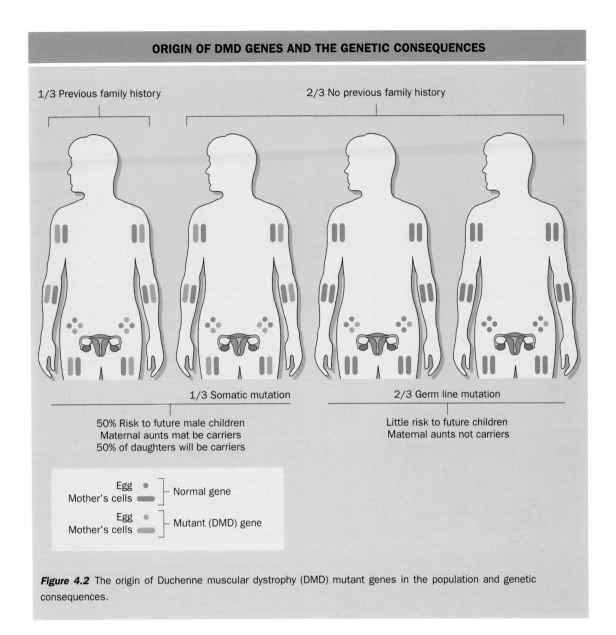

1/3 Previous family history   2/3 No previous family history

1/3 Somatic mutation   2/3 Germ line mutation

50% Risk to future male children
Maternal aunts mat be carriers
50% of daughters will be carriers

Little risk to future children
Maternal aunts not carriers

Egg
Mother's cells — Normal gene

Egg
Mother's cells — Mutant (DMD) gene

Figure 4.2 The origin of Duchenne muscular dystrophy (DMD) mutant genes in the population and genetic consequences.

(including where the maternal grandmother is a previously undiagnosed carrier) in about a third, while in the rest the mutation has occurred for the first time in the boys themselves (or to be more accurate in the ovum which produced them). The latter are so-called germ line mutations. The overall rate of new mutations within the general population is relatively high, at about 1 in 10,000.

In BMD, the frequency of new mutations is only about 10%. Males with BMD are usually able to have children, unlike boys with DMD. Thus the genetic defect is passed on through both male and female lines so that a greater proportion of mutations is inherited.

In DMD an affected male always results in the termination of that limb of a pedigree.

Once a diagnosis of DMD is made in a boy the rest of the family should be offered genetic counselling. This is particularly important for maternal aunts, who may be unwitting carriers of DMD. Counselling must be performed with sensitivity and tact. The responsibility of the clinician is to liase closely with the local clinical genetics service which has trained counsellors who can discuss the complex genetic and ethical issues with appropriate family members. Sadly, some families are still not offered genetic counselling until it is too late.

DIAGRAM OF THE CELL SURFACE AND CYTOSKELETAL PROTEIN COMPLEX

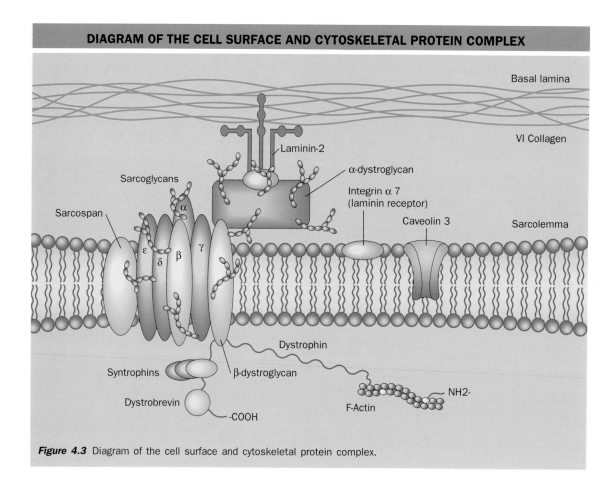

Figure 4.3 Diagram of the cell surface and cytoskeletal protein complex.

Molecular genetics

Dystrophin is a large protein, which localises to the sarcolemma on immunocytochemistry. It is part of a complex of proteins that link the intracellular cytoskeletal proteins including F-Actin to the extracellular matrix and is thought to impart structural integrity to the plasma membrane and to prevent contraction-induced damage. The other identified members of the complex are the sarcoglycans (α- = adhalin, β-, γ-, δ- and ε), the dystroglycans (α- and β-), the syntrophins (α-, β1- and β2-) and the laminins (α2- which is also known as merosin, β1- and γ1-) (Figure 4.3). Mutations of many of the genes for these proteins have already been implicated in the other dystrophies.

The gene for dystrophin lies on the X-chromosome at Xp21. It is very large, being 2500 KB long and consists of more than 70 exons. This accounts for the high mutation rate mentioned above. The commonest form of mutation is a deletion within the gene (65-70% of cases of DMD, over 80% of BMD), while 5-10% have duplications and the rest are assumed to have point mutations. There are certain "hot spots" for deletions and duplications where they are most likely to occur. These are principally in the first 20 exons and in the central region of the gene (exons 45-55). With a few exceptions, the clinical phenotype correlates poorly with the size of the deletion, but better with whether the deletion disrupts the nucleotide reading frame (i.e. whether they are "in-frame" or "out-of-frame" mutations). Mutations in certain areas of the gene are also associated with particular phenotypes. Thus relatively mild BMD is commonly associated with deletions in exons 45-47, while deletions in the proximal parts of the gene may be associated with severe myalgia and cramps rather than a typical dystrophy.

Clinical features

Duchenne dystrophy

Although DMD and BMD differ in severity, the clinical phenotype is otherwise remarkably similar in the two conditions. They are both characterised by progressive weakness and wasting of predominantly proximal musculature, but also involve distal muscles. Pseudohypertrophy of the calves, and more rarely other muscle groups is also seen (Figure 4.4).

In DMD, symptoms are always apparent by 5 years of age but commonly it is after the child begins to walk that the parents are aware of a problem. Not infrequently it takes them a long time to persuade the medical profession that there is anything wrong. There will have been an abnormal gait, frequent falls or simply the inability to keep up with their peers. In retrospect however the parents will recognise that motor development has been slow even before this. Fifty per cent or more of patients are unable to walk by the age 18 months and some do not walk even by the age of three years. At an earlier stage the child may have been noted to have prominent calves, to have been hypotonic or simply awkward. He may complain of pains in the muscles after exercise and myoglobinuria may occasionally occur.

On examination there is a striking selectivity of muscle involvement that tends to be symmetrical and predominantly affects the muscles of the limb girdle and proximal limb. Early on boys may just be able to rise from a sitting position without using their arms. As the weakness progresses this develops into the classical Gower's manoeuvre (Figure 4.5), which is the result of weakness of the extensors of the knee and hip. The gait becomes waddling in character due to weakness of the hip abductors and there is an accentuated lumbar lordosis due to weakness of the hip extensors. In the majority of cases accumulation of connective and adipose tissue results in pseudohypertrophy of the calves. On palpation these muscles have a characteristic "doughy" or "woody" consistency. A small number of patients have pseudohypertrophy of other muscles including the deltoids, masseters and even the tongue.

As the child becomes older, the weakness and wasting become more generalised. Sometimes there may be periods of apparent arrest, but usually the progression is fairly relentless. Intercurrent illness or periods of prolonged bed rest (for example following surgical procedures) may lead to a rapid deterioration in strength including the loss of ability to walk. Such periods of inactivity should therefore be avoided if possible. The tendency to walk on the toes may be associated with contractures of the Achilles' tendons. There is also a tendency towards and kyphoscoliosis, particularly after the patient becomes wheelchair bound. Active physiotherapy and spinal bracing may help to overcome this. If, however, thoracic deformities are allowed to develop they may in turn contribute to the progressive deterioration in pulmonary function and frequent chest infections.

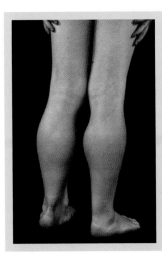

Figure 4.4
Duchenne muscular dystrophy. Calf pseudohypertrophy. (Courtesy of Dr Stephanie A Robb.)

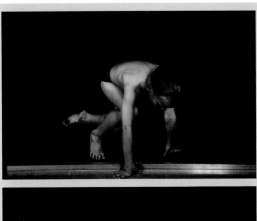

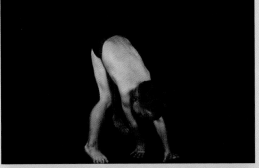

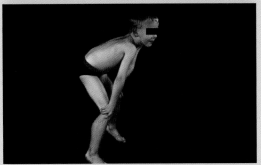

Figure 4.5 Gower's manoeuvre. (Courtesy of Dr Stephanie A Robb.)

Other tissues than muscle may be affected in Duchenne dystrophy, principally cardiac muscle and the brain. Characteristically there are ECG changes including tall R waves in the anterior chest leads with deep Q waves in the lateral chest leads and conduction defects. There may be cardiac murmurs, particularly of mitral valve prolapse, and asymptomatic sinus tachycardias are observed. Echocardiography shows abnormalities in about 50% of patients, but progressive cardiac failure occurs only very rarely before the terminal stages of the disease when respiratory failure complicates matters. It may be that with newer therapies, which extend lifespan in DMD, impairment of cardiac function becomes more important. Currently, however, cardiac dysfunction is of less practical importance in DMD than in many other myopathies.

There is evidence of global intellectual impairment in DMD. Many studies have shown a downward shift in the IQ distribution to about one standard deviation below the normal mean. Although some patients have high IQs, about 20% have an IQ of less than 70. These figures remain valid even when corrected for physical limitations and educational opportunities. Indeed the intellectual impairment is not progressive and is evident before muscle weakness is severe. There is also a difference between performance and verbal IQ with the latter being more profoundly affected. The verbal IQ deficit is mainly due to problems with verbal memory. Routine investigation with CT and MRI scanning has shown only minor cerebral atrophy, while post-mortem neuropathological studies have revealed only minor changes in dendritic development and microscopic heterotopias. These latter changes may, however, be the substrate for the intellectual changes seen. There is currently no convincing evidence of a specific correlation between the precise genetic abnormality and the degree of intellectual impairment.

Becker muscular dystrophy

Although BMD is in many ways a milder version of DMD there are some differences that are not merely of degree. The disease is more variable, but this is inevitable given the clinical definition of the disease compared to that of DMD (Table 4.2). While the typical age of onset of symptoms in BMD is between 5 and 15 years of age, it may be far later and patients may not present until their 30s or 40s. The selectivity of muscle involvement is similar to that in DMD and pseudohypertrophy is also common. Contractures and spinal deformity are uncommon, however, even in wheelchair bound patients.

The variability in the disorder is also manifest in relation to prognosis, which is far more difficult to assess than in DMD. In general patients with lower levels of dystrophin in muscle tend to have a more severe phenotype (such as "intermediate-type" dystrophinopathy), and patients with deletions at the N- or especially the C-terminal ends of the gene have a more severe clinical phenotype than those in the central rod domain. There is considerable clinical variability, however.

Intellectual impairment is very much less common in BMD than DMD, but it is becoming clear that a sizeable proportion of patients with BMD have cardiac involvement at relatively early stages of the disease. A dilated cardiomyopathy is the commonest serious manifestation and may occur in patients with very mild muscle weakness. It is also associated with the syndrome of myoglobinuria and cramps with dystrophinopathy. We recommend therefore that patients with BMD should have regular echocardiography since early intervention may improve long-term outlook, as is the case with other dilated cardiomyopathies.

Other dystrophinopathies

A number of other syndromes have been described that are associated with abnormalities of the dystrophin gene. They comprise a small but important group of disorders.

As already mentioned, female carriers of DMD or BMD may show clinically detectable muscle involvement (about 5-10% of patients) which is similar to that of typical male patients. This appears due to a skewed (non-random) pattern of X-chromosome inactivation resulting in a large proportion of fibres in muscle having defective dystrophin.

Patients with minimal muscle weakness and a syndrome of painful muscles with cramps (especially related to exercise) have been described in association with deletions within the dystrophin gene. They have occasional episodes of myoglobinuria. The CK is markedly and persistently elevated (10-100 times normal) in these patients. Other muscle manifestations associated with abnormal dystrophin include isolated elevations of CK and an isolated quadriceps myopathy.

In addition to the cardiomyopathy associated with DMD or BMD, there are reports of families and isolated patients in whom there is a significant dilated cardiomyopathy associated with a deletion of exon 1 of the dystrophin gene and of the muscle promoter region. This deletion modifies expression of dystrophin in a tissue-specific fashion with failure of expression only in cardiac muscle. Patients with an otherwise unexplained familial dilated cardiomyopathy should be screened for the deletion, especially if there is a suggestion of X-linked inheritance.

Diagnosis

The possibility of a patient having a dystrophinopathy is suggested by a typical history of motor problems suggestive of proximal weakness with appropriate signs as described previously. A high serum CPK and a myopathic EMG lend support to the diagnosis, although in a child one tries to avoid unnecessary use of needle EMG. For similar reasons, where the diagnosis of DMD or BMD can be made simply on genetic analysis of blood, muscle biopsy can and usually should be avoided.

In general it should be possible to detect large deletions or duplications within the dystrophin gene by straightforward genetic analysis. Thus 60-70% of patients with DMD and 80% of BMD patients are detectable without muscle biopsy. It is more difficult to detect point mutations or very small deletions in the

gene although novel techniques are being developed to try to overcome this problem. Sequencing the whole gene is not feasible at present since the gene is so large.

In this group of "deletion-negative" patients muscle biopsy and staining for dystrophin is required (Figure 4.6). The biopsy will show dystrophic changes with abnormal variation in fibre size. There are both very large and very small fibres, areas of focal necrosis and regenerating fibres and replacement of muscle fibres with fat and connective tissue. With dystrophin staining, there is complete absence of dystrophin in the surface membrane of myocytes in DMD (although occasional positive fibres – so-called revertant fibres – may be found), while in BMD the staining is usually reduced in intensity or is patchy, although in a few cases it may appear normal. In asymptomatic carriers, a mosaic pattern of staining (i.e. some normal and some negative or abnormally staining fibres – see Figure 4.6) may be seen but in most staining is normal. In young boys with a dystrophy the pattern of staining on

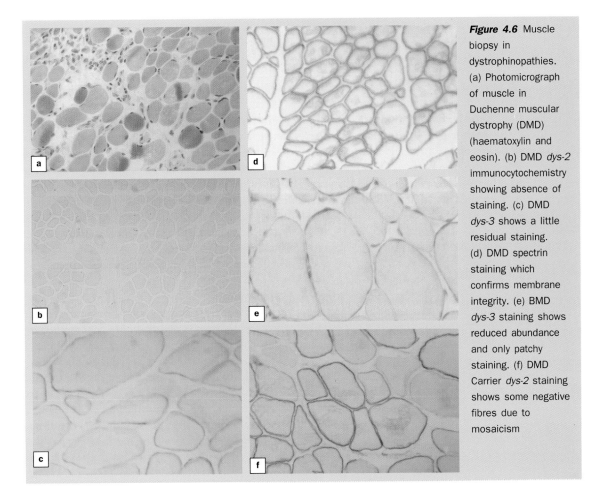

Figure 4.6 Muscle biopsy in dystrophinopathies. (a) Photomicrograph of muscle in Duchenne muscular dystrophy (DMD) (haematoxylin and eosin). (b) DMD *dys-2* immunocytochemistry showing absence of staining. (c) DMD *dys-3* shows a little residual staining. (d) DMD spectrin staining which confirms membrane integrity. (e) BMD *dys-3* staining shows reduced abundance and only patchy staining. (f) DMD Carrier *dys-2* staining shows some negative fibres due to mosaicism

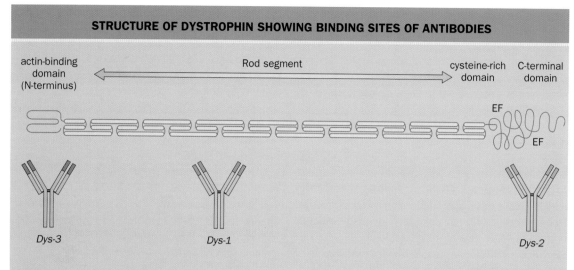

STRUCTURE OF DYSTROPHIN SHOWING BINDING SITES OF ANTIBODIES

Figure 4.7 Structure of dystrophin showing the binding sites of commercially available antibodies. More severe disease tends to result from loss of the C-terminal domain. In Figure 4.6 the child with DMD has no staining with *dys-2* but some with *dys-3* suggesting loss of the C-terminal domain.

immunohistochemistry may therefore provide some information which is useful in assessing prognosis.

There are three commonly used antibodies to the dystrophin molecule (to the C- and N-terminals and to the rod domain) and since truncated but non-functional proteins may be produced in affected individuals, it is important to use all three antibodies to confirm presence or absence of the protein (Figure 4.7). In addition, where muscle biopsy is used to check carrier status it is important to appreciate that some carriers of sarcoglycan-deficient limb girdle muscular dystrophy (see below) may show reduced dystrophin staining (without being carriers of a dystrophinopathy). Thus in this situation at least a full sarcoglycan panel must be tested as well.

In cases where staining is ambiguous then Western blotting (immunoblotting) to confirm reduced abundance of dystrophin in muscle is required or dystrophin of reduced molecular weight. This technique may also be useful in assessing carrier status in some potential female carriers of dystrophinopathies, but even this technique is not 100% effective. More refined genetic analysis including linkage analysis to areas within and close to the gene and more direct techniques such as in situ hybridization and DNA dosage analysis are then required.

Genetic counselling

Once the diagnosis is made, it is important to then consider the family as a whole and to embark upon genetic counselling. This is the process of ascertaining the risk of individuals within the family carrying, and then passing on the disease, and then conveying this and other useful information to them including the options available for reducing the risks of passing on the disease.

It follows that genetic counselling requires a broad knowledge of the disease under discussion, a sensitive approach to patients who will have very specific fears about themselves and their loved ones, as well as close collaboration with molecular genetic laboratories. All of this must be done in a "non-directive" fashion so that the patient and family are enabled to come to their own decisions about issues rather than having the counsellor's views imposed upon them. This means that genetic counselling requires special training and is not a task for the tyro or for the clinician without specific training.

Management

There are particular challenges in the management of patients with dystrophinopathies. Many of these relate to the coexistence of a progressive disorder and a growing child. The principles applying to physiotherapy and the orthopaedic management of patients with DMD are outlined in Chapter 3. The timing of surgery for contractures, and for the correction of scoliosis is a matter of very fine judgement and requires experience and close multidisciplinary planning.

The general considerations in the management of the patient with BMD are similar to those for DMD.

Progressive spinal deformities may affect those patients with a more aggressive form of BMD, or those with intermediate forms but are far less of a problem for the majority of patients with BMD. Careful monitoring of respiratory function is just as important and timely intervention can markedly improve both quality of life and its duration.

Cardiac involvement is more of an issue in BMD than DMD. This is in part because the background skeletal myopathy is more indolent and the cardiac effects have longer to make themselves apparent. Congestive heart failure is treated in the usual fashion and brady- or tachyarrhythmias sought and treated. Respiratory problems may worsen heart failure by putting strain on the right side of the heart and therefore must be dealt with aggressively. Where conventional therapy of cardiac failure fails, and the patient's skeletal muscle disease does not preclude it, cardiac transplantation should be considered.

There is evidence that the use of prednisolone in children with DMD slows the progression of disability although the mechanism is not clear. Although widely used in the United States, its use in the United Kingdom and Europe is still controversial and further clinical trials are planned.

Limb girdle muscular dystrophies

The advances in molecular diagnosis and nosology of muscle disease mean that to label a patient as having "limb-girdle muscular dystrophy" (LGMD) is no longer an accurate or adequate diagnosis. Once dystrophin analysis became available it was clear that as many as 30% of female patients labelled as having LGMD were in fact carriers of mutations in the dystrophin gene. Since that time a variety of specific forms of LGMD have been identified and, with a full diagnostic service including genetic information and protein analysis, the majority of cases can now be classified. Nevertheless, the classification of the limb-girdle muscular dystrophies (LGMDs) is always changing and the classification shown in Table 4.3 will rapidly be expanded.

Genetics and pathophysiology

The relative proportion of the individual LGMDs varies between different populations and different ages. The first to be clearly characterised were due to mutations in the sarcoglycan group of membrane proteins. These five glycoproteins are closely associated with dystrophin and, together with the dystroglycans,

Table 4.3 Classification of limb-girdle muscular dystrophy

Inheritance/ Classification	Gene localisation	Gene product
Autosomal Dominant		
• LGMD 1A	5q22.3-q31.3	Myotilin
• LGMD 1B	1q11-q21	Lamin A/C
• LGMD 1C	3p25	Caveolin
• LGMD 1D	7q	
Autosomal Recessive		
• LGMD 2A	15q15.1-q21.1	Calpain-3
• LGMD 2B	2p12-p14	Dysferlin
• LGMD 2C	13q12	γ-sarcoglycan
• LGMD 2D	17q21	α-sarcoglycan
• LGMD 2E	4q12	β-sarcoglycan
• LGMD 2F	5q33-q34	δ-sarcoglycan
• LGMD 2G	17q11-q12	Titin cap (telethonin)
• LGMD 2H	9q31-q33	
• LGMD 2I	19q13.3	
• LGMD 2J	2q31	Titin

link dystrophin to laminin A2 (merosin) and hence to the basal lamina (Figure 4.3). It is assumed that they play a crucial role in maintenance of membrane integrity. Usually loss or deficiency of one sarcoglycan leads to reduction in levels of the others, suggesting they form a single functional complex. Diseases associated with deficiency of α-, β-, γ- and δ-sarcoglycans have been described. Deficiency of ε-sarcoglycan has been associated with CNS disease (dystonia and myoclonus), but not neuromuscular disease.

The sarcoglycanopathies are certainly not the only forms of LGMD, however. Two other well-characterised forms of autosomal recessive LGMD have also been described (LGMD 2A and 2B) which are due to mutations within calpain-3 (a muscle-specific member of a calcium-dependent protease family) and dysferlin (a novel protein localised to the sarcolemma) respectively. There are also a number of families where a recessive LGMD localises to different genetic loci but the protein defect responsible has yet to be identified. Of the rarer autosomal dominant LGMDs, one (LGMD 1C) is associated with mutations in the gene for caveolin-3, a muscle-specific protein associated with dystrophin (but not closely linked with the dystrophin-glycoprotein complex) and which may be involved in cell signal transduction. Interestingly, LGMD1B is associated with mutations in the Lamin A/C gene on

Table 4.4 *Some phenotypic features of the commoner limb-girdle muscular dystrophies*

Disorder/Group	Laboratory	Clinical
Calpain deficiency LGMD2A	CK 7-80x N Myopathic biopsy with Type 1 predominance Normal dystrophin/ sarcoglycans Protein diagnosis by immunoblotting	Onset 2-40 years Predominant atrophy esp. of the posterior compartments Achilles' tendon contractures early Scapular winging Hip adductors spared Respiratory muscles affected Cardiac not affected
Dysferlinopathy LGMD2B	CK 10-100x N Dystrophic biopsy Reduced dysferlin immunostaining on biopsy CT scan shows gastrocnemius atrophy	Onset in late teens Mild phenotype Early inability to tiptoe Mainly lower limb (quads, psoas) Arms later, esp. biceps No systemic complications
Sarcoglycanopathy LGMD2C-F	CK high Biopsy shows loss of relevant sarcoglycan and variable loss of others	Often childhood onset Calf hypertrophy common Severity of disease variable Often quadriceps sparing Respiratory and cardiac involvement in severe disease
Lamin A/C associated LGMD1B	CK normal or slight rise Mildly myopathic biopsy	Onset 5-20 years Proximal lower limb onset Slow progression Upper limbs by 30's Cardiomyopathy with A-V block common (>60%)
Caveolin deficiency LGMD1C	CK 4-25x N Myopathic biopsy with reduced caveolin (NB: Reduced caveolin also in DMD)	Onset approx. 5 years Proximal weakness Calf hypertrophy Exercise-induced cramps Variable progression

chromosome 1q11-q21 as is autosomal dominant Emery-Dreifuss muscular dystrophy. The phenotypes are, however, quite different with LGMD1B not being associated with contractures. An autosomal dominant dilated cardiomyopathy and a form of familial partial lipodystrophy are also allelic with LGMD1B.

Clinical features

Given the marked genetic heterogeneity of this group of disorders, and the clinical diversity seen in the dystrophinopathies it is not surprising that there are a wide range of LGMD phenotypes. There are different patterns of muscle group involvement, different ages of onset and differing grades of severity. Some closely resemble Duchenne dystrophy and γ-sarcoglycanopathy was known previously as severe childhood autosomal recessive muscular dystrophy (SCARMD) reflecting its similar severity. Indeed the clinical similarity of many forms of LGMD to dystrophinopathies explains why many female manifesting carriers of DMD and BMD carried a diagnosis of LGMD before the advent of molecular genetic testing. By contrast, some patients with LGMD present with a very mild and very late onset proximal myopathy quite unlike dystrophinopathy. The phenotypes associated with the different genetic entities are summarised in Table 4.4.

Diagnosis

The diagnosis of LGMD requires the clinical picture of a progressive proximal myopathy, with changes on investigation suggestive of a dystrophic process (variation in fibre size, fibre necrosis, increased intercellular connective tissue) and normal staining for dystrophin on muscle biopsy. (In recent years however some cases of sarcoglycan deficiency have been reported with (secondary) abnormal dystrophin staining. Usually the clinical severity is far greater than explicable on the basis of mild changes in dystrophin). A positive family history may enable classification into either autosomal dominant or autosomal recessive disease (and so into the broad groups of type 1 or 2 LGMD). Further studies using molecular genetic and muscle immunocytochemical testing may allow precise genetic characterisation of the disorder into one of the groups in Table 4.4. A particular feature to note is that while deficiency of one sarcoglycan may lead to secondary deficiency of the others, it is not invariably the case and for diagnostic security antibodies to all the sarcoglycans should be used in confirming a diagnosis of LGMD 2C-2F.

In addition to the disorders specifically called limb-girdle muscular dystrophies, a number of other dystrophies present as a predominantly limb girdle syndrome. These include the dystrophinopathies, Emery-Dreifuss muscular dystrophy, Bethlem myopathy, and congenital muscular dystrophies. Some of the "ultrastructural myopathies" such as desmin-storage myopathies, cytoplasmic body myopathy and myopathies with tubular aggregates present similarly and need to be considered in the differential diagnosis.

Management

The principles of management of the limb girdle dystrophies are the same as those for other dystrophies such as DMD or BMD and the general principles outlined in Chapter 3. Wherever possible an accurate genetic diagnosis should be sought, both for adequate genetic counselling but also because the individual genetic diseases have differing prognoses and complications.

Facioscapulohumeral muscular dystrophy

Facioscapulohumeral muscular dystrophy (FSH dystrophy) is an autosomal dominant dystrophy predominantly affecting the face, the serratus anterior and humeral muscles and the anterior tibial muscles. In its classical form it is very easy to recognise and diagnose.

It is, however, extremely variable in its severity even within families and under these circumstances can still provide a diagnostic challenge. The quoted prevalence figures vary widely, perhaps due the very mild nature of the disease in many subjects. The best estimates available are of a prevalence of 1.5–3 per 100,000. Molecular genetic analyses in families suggest that at least 10% of cases are due to new pathogenic mutations.

Genetics and pathophysiology

The disease is inherited in an autosomal dominant fashion and therefore is inherited by both sexes equally. There is however a difference in the degree of clinical penetrance so that female carriers of the gene have a somewhat later age of symptomatic presentation than do males (by the age of 30, 90% of males have symptoms but only 70% of females). Many patients have no symptoms even when clinical signs are clearly present if searched for. Physical signs are present at the age of 20 in 95% of cases, and in half of cases by the age of 15. It must be stressed, however, that these signs may be subtle, and that only after a careful and rigorous examination of muscle strength (and, now, genetic testing) is it possible to rule out the disorder. In asymptomatic cases, EMG and measurement of serum CK levels are not reliable in excluding the diagnosis. The EMG is only abnormal in about 50% of all patients (and may be normal in significantly affected patients) and CK is often normal. Even muscle biopsy often shows only minor myopathic changes although there is some evidence that biopsies of supraspinatus may have a greater diagnostic yield.

Molecular genetic testing is now available for the majority (95%) of affected families. The gene locus for FSHD in these families is on chromosome 4 (4q35). The region affected in the disease contains a numbers of repeats of a 3.3kb tandem repeat sequence which is guanine and cytosine (GC)-rich and contains two homeobox gene units. After digestion using EcoRI, DNA from normal subjects produces a fragment of 50 to 300kb, but in FSH patients the fragment size is 10-34kb due to loss of some DNA (Figure 4.8). One problem is that there is another area on chromosome 10 which shows 98-100% homology to 4q35 and which produces a similar fragment on EcoRI digestion. In 10% of normal subjects, the chromosome 10 fragments are less than 35kb thus leaving a diagnostic problem. To overcome this problem of false positive results that may result, a second DNA digestion is performed using the restriction enzyme BlnI. This digests only the chromosome 10 fragments and leaves the chromosome 4

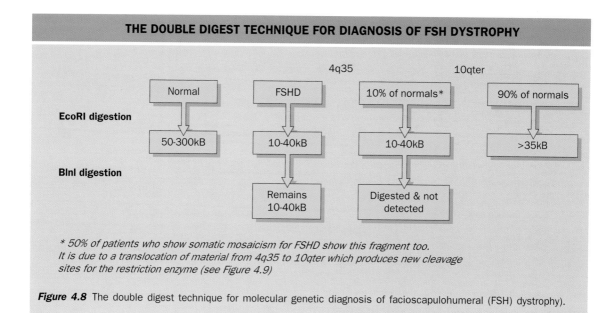

THE DOUBLE DIGEST TECHNIQUE FOR DIAGNOSIS OF FSH DYSTROPHY

* 50% of patients who show somatic mosaicism for FSHD show this fragment too. It is due to a translocation of material from 4q35 to 10qter which produces new cleavage sites for the restriction enzyme (see Figure 4.9)

Figure 4.8 The double digest technique for molecular genetic diagnosis of facioscapulohumeral (FSH) dystrophy.

GENETIC ABNORMALITIES IN FSH DYSTROPHY

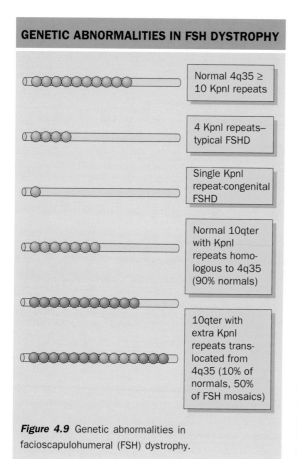

Figure 4.9 Genetic abnormalities in facioscapulohumeral (FSH) dystrophy.

fragments intact for diagnostic testing (Figures 4.8 & 4.9). This "double digest" test allows a diagnostic sensitivity and specificity each of 95%. No genes are known to be expressed from the abnormal region and it is assumed that the repeat sequence modifies the expression of neighbouring genes indirectly and that mutations therefore alter expression of one or more of these genes which is responsible for causing the disease.

There is a general relationship between the size of the DNA deletion and the severity of the disease (Figure 4.9). Thus the largest deletions (10-11kb residual fragments) tend to be associated with severe, congenital disease (while mothers may be somatic mosaics and minimally affected), while the smallest are sometimes associated with a scapulo-peroneal syndrome and may not be penetrant by 20 years old.

Clinical features

Although variable, the commonest age of onset of symptoms is between 7 and 30 years old. In about 65% of cases the initial presentation is asymmetrical, and the unwary clinician may suspect a neurogenic cause for early signs such as poliomyelitis or even a polyradiculopathy. In general the order in which clinically detectable weakness occurs is not the order in which the patient develops symptoms. Thus clinical examination reveals that after facial weakness, there is weakness of the dorsiflexors of the foot and the lower abdominal

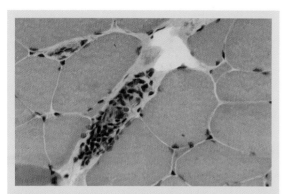

Figure 4.10 Muscle biopsy pathology in facioscapulohumeral dystrophy. Mildly myopathic appearance with a focus of inflammatory cells.

der girdle (often in the mid teens), weakness develops in triceps and biceps and eventually also of supraspinatus and the sternocostal head of pectoralis major. This latter feature gives rise to a pectoral fold that is characteristic of FSHD although not specific to it. Clinical features are shown in Figure 4.10.

Occasionally it is weakness of eye closure that brings the patient to seek medical help, often from an ophthalmologist, but the vast majority of patients present because of problems using the arms. The weakness of scapular fixation results in impairment of shoulder abduction beyond a certain angle. This is because although it is possible to achieve 90° of abduction using supraspinatus and deltoid, to go beyond this requires the scapula to be fixed to the chest wall. Thus in FSH dystrophy working above the head, or even combing hair may become impossible. Some patients develop trick movements to essentially fling the arm above the head and then use the other arm to support it and this sometimes delays their presentation further.

Symptomatic involvement of lower limb muscles occurs later in the disease but weakness of tibialis anterior (and sometimes the peroneii) can be demonstrated clinically in most patients early on. In a about half of patients the lower limb weakness is sufficient to cause symptoms. In a smaller proportion, weakness extends beyond the anterior and peroneal compartments to involve the pelvic girdle. In general this is associated with a poorer prognosis. Overall 19% of patients require a wheelchair by the time they are 40 years old but in general the prognosis in FSHD is good.

muscles, then the shoulder girdle and humeral muscles (usually sparing deltoid) and later on (in some) the pelvic girdle and proximal lower limb muscles. Contractures and scoliosis are rare.

In taking the history of symptoms, typically facial weakness is present first (although rarely volunteered as a symptom), and often the first sign is an inability to close the eyes tightly so that the patient is unable to bury his/her eyelids. The transverse smile and failure to be able to whistle that are also due to facial weakness are often considered family traits. This is also true of the odd shoulder contour (Figure 4.11) due to scapular winging from weakness of serratus anterior, the rhomboids and the lower part of trapezius. After weakness of the shoul-

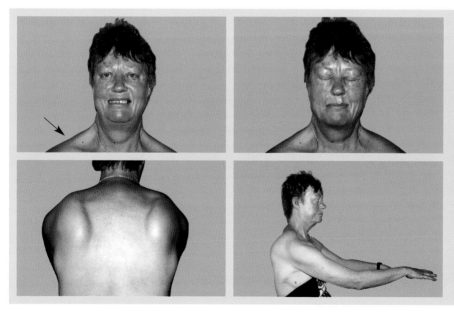

Figure 4.11 Clinical features of facioscapulohumeral dystrophy. (a) Facial appearance with a transverse smile and rather high riding scapulae (arrow). (b) Weakness of eye closure and asymmetric facial weakness. (c) Scapular winging. (d) On attempting to raise the arms, there is increased scapular winging

In 75% of cases there is evidence of high tone sensorineural hearing loss, but this is rarely severe enough to cause clinical problems. Similarly as many as 50 % of patients have changes of a retinal vasculopathy, with capillary telangectasis, microaneurysms, retinal oedema or haemorrhages on fluoroscein angiography but very few become symptomatic.

A common, but under-recognised problem in FSH dystrophy is pain, particularly around the shoulder girdle and upper arms. It may only be mentioned if the patient is directly questioned, but is nevertheless often described as disabling. Although some pain is due to abnormal posture secondary to weakness, much of the pain is myalgic in nature. The origin of this pain is unclear but specific causes such as glenohumeral dislocation should be excluded before embarking upon non-specific treatments.

Congenital FSH dystrophy

In a small proportion of cases changes of FSH dystrophy are present from birth. These cases have more severe involvement, often with complete bilateral facial palsy which itself provides a significant social handicap for a young child since they are unable to smile. Limb weakness tends to develop more rapidly and many affected children require a wheelchair by the time they are 20. A degree of mental retardation may also occur and epilepsy is commoner than in the general population. It is associated with the largest DNA deletions.

Diagnosis

In the majority of cases the diagnosis of FSH dystrophy is clear once it has occurred to the examining clinician. There is a differential diagnosis (Table 4.5) but the alert clinician should not often be caught out. Genetic testing generally confirms diagnosis and helps subsequent genetic counselling. Muscle biopsy is necessary only where there is diagnostic doubt and where genetic testing has proved unhelpful while EMG studies, as already mentioned are not helpful.

Table 4.5 *Differential diagnosis of facioscapulohumeral muscular dystrophy*

Facioscapulohumeral muscular dystrophy (FSH dystrophy)

Myotonic dystrophy

Limb-girdle muscular dystrophies (esp. LGMD 2A)

Centronuclear myopathy

Nemaline myopathy

Other scapuloperoneal syndromes (see Table 4.6)

Syndromes of absent muscles

Muscle biopsy

For maximum information, as in all myopathies, it is important that a muscle that is clinically affected is biopsied. It must not, however, be too severely affected. The slow progress of FSH dystrophy and the selectivity of muscle involvement mean that biopsies often show only marginal and non-specific changes.

In well-developed disease, there is evidence of myopathic change with an increase in fibre size variability. The average size of the fibres is increased but scattered throughout the biopsy are small angulated fibres. Some regenerating fibres are seen, although less than in dystrophinopathies, and there are some fibres containing internal nuclei and a mild and variable increase in endomysial connective tissue. Perhaps the most unusual feature of FSH dystrophy is the degree of inflammation seen in biopsies. Focal areas of mononuclear cell infiltrates are seen in the majority of cases either scattered in the perimysium or in a perivascular distribution (Figure 4.10).

Management

No specific treatment exists for FSH dystrophy. Despite the frequent inflammatory infiltrates on muscle biopsy, prednisolone therapy is ineffective. Other agents have been studied but none have yet been shown to be effective.

Non-specific treatments include the provision of foot-drop splints where involvement of tibialis anterior is severe and the provision of analgesics and physiotherapy for pain.

For patients who are significantly impaired by inability to raise their arms above their head, scapular fixation may provide improved mechanical function if the deltoid muscle remains strong. The operation tends to be painful, however, and results (as judged by the patient) are quite variable. Most patients do not opt for surgery.

Scapuloperoneal syndromes, including scapuloperoneal muscular dystrophy

Scapuloperoneal muscular dystrophy is only one of the causes of a scapuloperoneal syndrome (Table 4.6). The syndrome is quite rare and the various causes can be extremely similar clinically. Sometimes only special investigations will allow differential diagnosis. Electromyography may allow differentiation between the neuropathic, neuronopathic (anterior horn cell) and

Table 4.6 *Scapuloperoneal syndromes without 4q35 linkage*

Scapuloperoneal muscular dystrophy

Emery-Dreifuss dystrophy

Davidenkow's syndrome (scapuloperoneal neuropathy)

Centronuclear myopathy (adult onset)

Mitochondrial (including FSH phenotype with ragged red fibers & cardiomyopathy)

Acid maltase deficiency with scapuloperoneal weakness

Limb-girdle dystrophy (LGMD) 2A

Scapuloperoneal neuronopathy

Late onset reducing body myopathy

myopathic causes of the scapuloperoneal syndrome. Occasionally, however, the muscle biopsy findings are not those expected from the EMG and muscle biopsy should be performed in all cases. Biopsy will then allow differentiation of the various myopathic causes or confirmation of neurogenic change. When analysis suggests a dystrophy, clinical assessment should have excluded Emery-Dreifuss muscular dystrophy and a close examination for facial involvement and genetic analysis should be carried out to exclude FSH dystrophy as a cause.

Scapuloperoneal muscular dystrophy (SPMD) in its pure form is usually dominantly inherited with about 60-80% penetrance. The gene localises to chromosome 12q13.3-15. Onset is usually in the third to sixth decades and may occur in the legs with foot drop or in the arms with shoulder weakness. Scapular winging is common and asymmetry, similar to that seen in FSH dystrophy may be seen. Some patients show a rapid progression of symptoms but in most progression is slow and life expectancy unaffected.

Investigation of patients with SPMD reveals a mild to moderate rise in CK (1.5-10 times normal) while biopsy shows patchy myopathic change, sometimes with eosinophilic inclusions (most commonly in type I fibres) that stain positively for desmin.

A quite separate X-linked scapuloperoneal muscular dystrophy with onset at about 5 years of age and death in the second or third decade has also been described. It is associated with hypertrophic cardiomyopathy, mental retardation and myopia. Carriers may develop hypertrophic cardiomyopathy.

Scapuloperoneal peripheral neuropathy (Davidenkow's syndrome) is an autosomal dominant condition whose age of onset varies widely. Weakness usually appears first in the distal legs followed by the shoulder girdle. There is pes cavus and progressive distal sensory loss, which differentiates it from myopathic causes of a scapuloperoneal syndrome. Ankle jerks are absent and other reflexes are sluggish. Nerve conduction studies show an axonal neuropathy with absent sensory potentials.

Scapuloperoneal neuronopathy (motor neuron disease) occurs in a number of forms with autosomal dominant and recessive inheritance described in different families. In one dominant form linked to chromosome 12q24.1-q24.31 there is congenital absence of muscles and a progressive scapuloperoneal and distal weakness with laryngeal palsy.

Emery–Dreifuss muscular dystrophy

The crucial importance of Emery–Dreifuss dystrophy (DMS) is that there is an extremely high incidence of cardiac involvement that, if unrecognised, may lead to conduction block, arrhythmias and sudden death (in more than 40% of cases).

Genetics and pathophysiology
Emery-Dreifuss dystrophy is usually inherited as an X-linked recessive disorder, although several families with an almost identical clinical picture showing autosomal dominant inheritance have been described. In the X-linked form there is 100% penetrance by the third decade of life. Female carriers generally show no evidence of a myopathy, but cardiac rhythm disturbances may be observed. It is suggested that carriers be kept under careful cardiac review.

The gene responsible is located at the extreme end of the long arm of the X chromosome (Xq28). It is very small (<2kb long) and codes a novel 34kD protein, emerin that localises to the inner nuclear membrane of muscle (skeletal and cardiac) and in the cytoplasm of other cell types. The physiological role of emerin is unknown. A wide variety of mutations have been described in the gene all of which result in either absence or reduced abundance of emerin in the muscle nuclear membrane.

Clinical features
The onset of symptoms is usually at about 4-5 years old. EMD is characterised by a triad of features consisting of (1) early development of contractures of the elbows, posterior neck and Achilles' tendons – often before there is significant weakness, (2) a humeroperoneal distribution of weakness initially, later involving proximal limb girdle muscles and (3) cardiac involvement

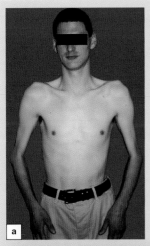

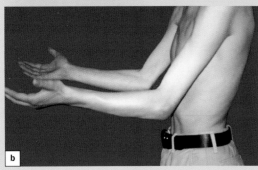

Figure 4.12
Emery–Dreifuss muscular dystrophy. (a) Scapulohumeral distribution of wasting. There is a scar from pacemaker insertion. (b) Fixed flexion contractures at the elbow (also obvious in (a))

The diagnosis of X-linked EMD may be confirmed either by muscle or skin biopsy. Muscle biopsies show a dystrophic pattern of changes (necrotic and regenerating fibres, variation in fibre size, increased internal nuclei) but no specific changes. Immunocytochemistry for emerin shows absent or reduced staining.

Skin biopsies may also be used for diagnosis and also for carrier ascertainment. In the latter instance skewed X-inactivation may mean that levels of emerin on Western blotting and on staining of a muscle biopsy are normal. Skin biopsies are more reliable in that some emerin-negative nuclei are always observed in carriers although for best results two separate skin biopsies should be examined.

Management

The most important specific aspect of management is cardiac follow up and insertion of a pacemaker where appropriate. Although pacing may be life saving, only the conduction block is relieved and later on in the disease the progressive cardiomyopathy may be life threatening. Under these circumstances, patients may be considered for cardiac transplantation.

Physiotherapy with active and passive muscle stretching may help to slow down the development of contractures although, since they develop early, prevention is difficult. Some patients will require Achilles tenotomies.

Bethlem myopathy

Bethlem myopathy is an autosomal dominant myopathy that is not normally classified as a muscular dystrophy, but does not easily fit into other groups such as the congenital myopathies. We consider it here for completeness and because of its importance as a differential diagnosis for some of the dystrophies such as Emery-Dreifuss and some forms of LGMD.

Onset is in early life, with some mothers having noted reduced foetal movements. The newborn may be hypotonic and other childhood cases present before the age of 2. There is diffuse and mild proximal weakness, sometimes causing falls and some cases improve in early childhood, and most around puberty. In adult life, however, the weakness may return in the 3rd-5th decades and many become wheelchair bound in their 50s or 60s.

There is a striking tendency to contractures in many but not all families. These frequently affect the hands with flexion deformities of the interphalangeal joints of the fingers, as well as the wrists, elbows and ankles. The

with atrioventricular conduction block. The contractures produce a characteristic appearance when fully developed (Figure 4.12) but in the early stages should be actively sought. As weakness develops there is an increased lumbar lordosis and a waddling gait. There is an increased risk of malignant hyperpyrexia.

Even in those in whom muscle weakness is minimal there may be severe cardiac involvement. Atrioventricular conduction is usually impaired with sinus bradycardia, various degrees of heart block atrial flutter and fibrillation. Atrial paralysis may occur and in apparently isolated atrial paralysis (i.e. without overt cardiac or skeletal muscle disease) mutations in the emerin gene are common. Later in the course of the disease a more generalised cardiomyopathy with congestive heart failure may develop.

Diagnosis

The diagnosis must be considered in any patient presenting with a humero-peroneal syndrome, and especially if contractures are present early in the disease. An abnormal ECG will often provide the major clue to diagnosis.

patient is unable to put the hands flat together (as if praying). Contractures may also affect the shoulders, knees or hips. Unlike Emery-Dreifuss dystrophy, which is a major differential diagnosis, there is no cardiac involvement.

Diagnosis is clinical, with only non-specific changes on muscle biopsy (including variation in fibre size, splitting, and increased internal nucleation), a myopathic EMG and frequently normal CK levels. Mutations in various subunits of collagen VI, one component of the basement membrane are responsible .

Myotonic dystrophy

Myotonic dystrophy (dystrophia myotonica, DM1) is the commonest adult muscular dystrophy (lifetime incidence at least 1 in 8,000) and is characterised by early distal muscle weakness and wasting, failure of muscle relaxation (myotonia) and a number of clinically important and potentially serious non-muscular manifestations affecting the heart, eye and central nervous system in particular. Although traditionally classified together with the non-dystrophic myotonias, the genetic and pathophysiological basis is quite different from the channelopathies and it is more properly classified with the other dystrophies.

Genetics
Myotonic dystrophy (DM1) is inherited as an autosomal dominant disorder, but the phenotype has long been known to be extremely variable. It was noted as long ago as the 1940s that the disease seems to occur at younger ages and with greater severity in successive generations of an affected family. This phenomenon is known as anticipation. Initially it was considered that this may merely reflect ascertainment bias but elucidation of the genetic basis of the disease has provided evidence of a genetic basis for anticipation. At its most severe, the child of a minimally affected mother may be severely affected from birth (congenital myotonic dystrophy – see below).

DM1 is associated with an increased number of repeats of the trinucleotide sequence cytosine, thymine and guanine (CTG) in the 3'-untranslated region of a gene on chromosome 19. This gene codes for a protein, myotonin protein kinase (MT-PK), which is widely expressed in a number of tissues but whose function is as yet unclear. In normal individuals there are between 5 and 30 repeats of the CTG trinucleotide (but the commonest number is 5, 11 or 12 repeats). In patients with myotonic dystrophy

Table 4.7 A comparison of some features of classical and type 2 myotonic dystrophy

	DM1	DM2
Age at onset	Any	8 to 50 years
Clinical anticipation	+	±
Weakness		
Face	+	+
Ptosis	+	±
Proximal	±	+
Distal	+	+
Sternomastoid	+	Variable
Cardiac arrhythmias	+	+
Cataracts	+	+
Hypersomnia	+	Variable
Frontal balding	+	+
Hypogonadism	+	Variable
Insulin resistance	+	Variable
Calf hypertrophy	-	+
Hyperhidrosis	Variable	+
Electromyogram: myotonia	+	+
Gene locus	19q13.3	3q21

there are more than 50 repeats in those minimally affected and sometimes over 2,000 repeats in severely affected individuals (including congenital MyD). In very general terms the larger the repeat number, the more severe is the disease and the earlier the onset of symptoms. The way in which the mutation in an untranslated area of the MT-PK gene causes the clinical phenotype of myotonic dystrophy is still not entirely clear.

A few families have been described that have a disorder almost indistinguishable from classical myotonic dystrophy, but in whom there is no evidence of a CTG expansion. Some families show linkage to a locus on chromosome 3, but in others there is no linkage either to the MT-PK locus on chromosome 19 or to the chromosome 3 locus. This condition, with linkage to chromosome 3, has been named DM2 (whereas classical myotonic dystrophy is DM1) and a comparison of the two conditions is shown in Table 4.7. Proximal myotonic myopathy (PROMM, see below) also links to the same, or a very close locus on chromosome 3 and is allelic with DM2.

Clinical features
The major clinical features of classical myotonic dystrophy (DM1) are shown in Table 4.8. Those considered of particular clinical importance are considered further below.

Table 4.8 *Major clinical features of myotonic dystrophy (DM1)*

Skeletal muscle
- Weakness & wasting
  - Distal > Proximal
  - More generalised later in disease
  - Neck muscles especially affected
  - Facial weakness & ptosis
  - Weakness may be disproportionate to wasting
- Myotonia
  - Present on voluntary contraction (e.g. grip) and percussion of muscle
  - Sometimes worsened by cold
  - May affect jaw, tongue, palate causing dysarthria
  - Rarely a major cause of disability

Heart
- Conduction block
- Atrial & ventricular arrhythmias
- Increased incidence of sudden cardiac death
- Mitral valve prolapse (common but benign)
- Dilating cardiomyopathy (rare)

Eye
- Early lens opacities
- Cataract
- Ptosis
- Retinal pigmentary change (rare)

CNS
- Hypersomnolence
- Apathetic personality trait
- Low average IQ

Integument
- Frontal balding (most marked in men)
- Association with multiple pilomatrixomata

Smooth muscle
- Oesophagus (dysphagia)
- Colon (constipation, colic, faecal soiling)
- Gallbladder (higher incidence of stones at younger age)
- Uterus (tendency to poor labour)

Endocrine
- Testicular tubular atrophy
- Peripheral insulin resistance
- Hyperresponsiveness of insulin to a glucose load (NB: Clinical diabetes mellitus uncommon)

Skeletal muscle

The most obvious clinical features are to be found in skeletal muscle. The myotonia from which the disease derives its name is the result of sustained contraction of muscle due to abnormal repetitive electrical activity of the muscle membrane. It may be seen on voluntary contraction (usually on gripping the examiners fingers) and by percussion of certain muscles, particularly the abductor pollicis brevis or the long finger extensors (see Chapter 1). Myotonia of the mouth and pharynx may cause dysarthria or dysphagia. Myotonia is sometimes worsened by cold (although this is far commoner in myotonia due to sodium channelopathies) and tends to be reduced by repeated contraction of the muscle (the so-called "warm-up" phenomenon). It is rarely a major problem to the patient, however. This is unlike the non-dystrophic myotonias such as myotonia congenita (Chapter 6) where myotonia can cause significant disability.

A greater problem to the patient than myotonia is muscular weakness. In the early stages of the disease this usually affects the distal forearms causing weak grip and may be out of proportion to any myotonia or wasting of the muscle (for reasons that are unclear). The muscles around the neck are also affected early on in the disease with prominent wasting and weakness of the sternomastoid muscles. Facial weakness and wasting result in the long haggard facies associated with the condition (Figure 4.13) and ptosis is common. Foot drop is also common in early disease with a tendency to trip and fall. As the disease progresses the weakness becomes more generalised but the predominantly distal pattern of weakness is still retained.

Cardiac function

The heart is very commonly involved in both types of myotonic dystrophy and heart block represents the major *treatable* complication of the disease. It may occur even in patients with relatively mild muscular manifestations so that active cardiac management is required even in minimally symptomatic individuals. Prospective studies show a high incidence of ECG abnormalities (in 30-80% of all patients) while cohort studies show a progressive increase in PR and QRS intervals in most patients studied. These changes are predictable and gradual, however, so that regular follow-up should identify early those patients who will require pacemaker insertion. There is also a tendency to develop both atrial and paroxysmal ventricular tachyarrythmias, and sudden death is more common in DM1 than in the general population. There are usually no warning signs of ventricular dysrhythmias on surface ECG between episodes but careful questioning about syncopal attacks or palpitations will identify a group who require more thorough cardiac assessment with 24-hour Holter monitoring. Symptomatic myocardial

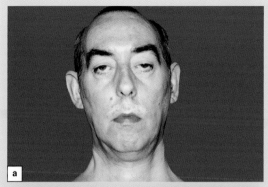

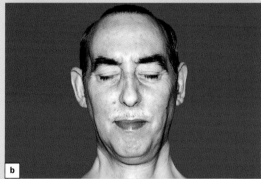

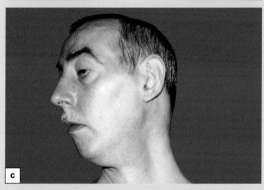

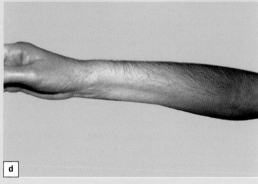

Figure 4.13 Myotonic dystrophy (DM1). (a) Facial appearance. (b) Weakness of eye closure. (c) Typical wasting of sternocleidomastoid. (d) Forearm flexor compartment wasting.

involvement with myocarditis and dilated cardiomyopathy occurs but is rare.

Central nervous system
About 40% of patients with DM1 have some degree of intellectual impairment and it is a particular feature of the congenital form. In addition many patients display a rather characteristic personality type with general lethargy, apathy and a lack of drive. There is also a marked tendency to hypersomnolence, which may be so severe that a patient will admit to having slept through the whole day. This feature is seen even in very mildly affected patients and, although respiratory failure may play a role in a few patients, in the majority there is a central cause.

Ocular manifestations
Lens changes are almost universal in DM1 and in mild cases may be the only clinical feature. Before genetic testing became available they were one of the markers used for the diagnosis of myotonic dystrophy. The earliest changes are only observable on slit-lamp examination and consist of iridescent multicoloured crystalline specks ("polychromatic dots") found in the posterior subcapsular region of the lens. These progress to form mature cataracts that are indistinguishable from senile cataracts. Extraocular muscles are usually not symptomatically affected by the disease although careful analysis of eye movements does reveal deficits in many patients. These deficits are thought to be central in origin, however, and rarely result in any clinical problem.

Smooth muscle
Although the brunt of symptoms fall upon skeletal and cardiac muscle, symptoms due to smooth muscle involvement are common. In particular dysphagia due to oesophageal dysmotility and colic or constipation due to colonic involvement are frequent complaints. Many patients have symptoms consistent with irritable bowel syndrome and there is an increased incidence of biliary tract dysfunction and gallstones.

Impaired function of uterine smooth muscle, combined with skeletal muscle weakness affecting abdominal muscles, results in a relatively high incidence of failure to progress in labour.

Endocrine features
Experimental studies on patients with DM1 have shown evidence of peripheral insulin resistance and hyperresponsiveness of insulin to a glucose load or

glucagon challenge. Nevertheless clinical diabetes mellitus is uncommon in myotonic dystrophy and we do not routinely screen patients for glucose intolerance in the absence of suggestive symptoms.

Testicular atrophy was noted in the very first descriptions of the disease and appears to result from atrophy of seminiferous tubules. Probably as a result of this, levels of FSH are often raised in males while those of LH are only marginally elevated.

Congenital myotonic dystrophy

This is a clearly recognisable subgroup of the disease occurring only in infants born to affected mothers with DM1 (not to the partners of affected males). It should not be confused with myotonia congenita, which is a non-dystrophic disorder. The features of congenital myotonic dystrophy are outlined in Table 4.9.

Frequently the affected child will be born to a mother in whom the diagnosis of myotonic dystrophy has not been made thus requiring considerable clinical vigilance on the part of the paediatrician. The pregnancy will often have been complicated by polyhydramnios and the mother may have noticed reduced movements. About a third of children have neonatal respiratory distress and many of these require ventilation. They are noted to be floppy infants and talipes or multiple contractures ("arthrogryposis") may be present at birth. The children have a characteristic bilateral facial weakness that results in a V-shaped tented upper lip (Figure 4.14) which, together with jaw weakness, causes difficulty feeding. If they survive the neonatal period they usually show mental retardation and

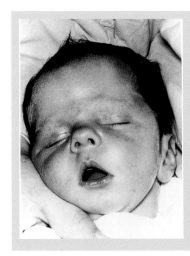

Figure 4.14 Picture of child with congenital myotonic dystrophy.

delayed motor milestones. Interestingly, however, clinical myotonia is not present at birth and frequently does not develop for years afterwards.

As indicated above, often the mother is only very mildly affected clinically although careful examination will reveal clinical myotonia in most cases. Indeed the diagnosis is usually made from examining the mother rather than the infant.

Diagnosis and Screening

In many cases the diagnosis is obvious on clinical grounds from the features of grip myotonia, distal weakness with wasting and the characteristic facial appearance. In such cases the only special investigation other than genetic testing that is mandatory is a 12-lead ECG to check for heart block or obvious arrhythmias. In other cases, and when screening a family for the disease further investigation is required. Since the discovery of the genetic defect this has been very simply performed by genetic analysis on leucocyte DNA derived from peripheral blood. Muscle biopsy has no part to play in diagnosis and electromyography (EMG) is only relevant if it reveals typical myotonic discharges in unsuspected cases in which the diagnosis is no more specific than "a myopathy" and have therefore undergone EMG.

Because of the potential for serious anaesthetic and cardiac complications in minimally symptomatic patients, as well as the risks of passing the disease on to children, screening should be offered to all individuals at risk of myotonic dystrophy. As with all pre-symptomatic testing, patients should be counselled about the consequences of undergoing testing (e.g. for future insurance, the consequences of a positive test etc.)

Table 4.9 Features of congenital myotonic dystrophy

Bilateral facial & jaw weakness
Hypotonia ("floppy infant")
Neonatal respiratory distress
Mental retardation
Delayed motor development
Talipes
Feeding difficulties
Lack of clinical myotonia
(Polyhydramnios)
(Reduced foetal movements)
Almost always mother-child transmission of DM gene
Associated with the largest trinucleotide repeat expansions

either for clinical or DNA testing, and screening should only be carried out on those capable of giving valid informed consent (i.e. adults).

Management

All aspects of the myotonic dystrophy may call for follow up but it is particularly important that patients receive annual review with a 12-lead ECG looking for progressive conduction defects. If there is significant heart block then pacing is indicated. The patient should also be questioned for symptoms of syncope and palpitations and if these are present then a 24-hour Holter ECG should be performed.

Drugs do not help the myopathic weakness that is the most significant complaint, although physiotherapy may be helpful and simple measures such as providing an ankle support can produce marked functional improvement. The surgical correction of troublesome ptosis is also sometimes indicated although attention must be paid to potential anaesthetic complications when deciding whether to recommend such surgery.

Myotonia is rarely a problem to the patient, but in the small number of cases in whom it is drug treatment may be helpful. Phenytoin and procainamide are the two most commonly used drugs although both should be used with caution in anyone with an abnormal ECG or cardiac symptoms. Nifedipine may also help in some cases. Mexilitene, which is helpful in myotonia associated with channelopathies, has also been used in a small number of patients with DM1. However, in view of its cardiac effects it should be used with great care and avoided unless there is disabling myotonia unresponsive to other agents.

More of a problem is excessive daytime somnolence. Frequently this will lead to major social handicap and stress within family relationships, where the sufferer is merely thought to be lazy – in keeping with the demeanour that they frequently portray. Central stimulants seem to have a role in treatment although controlled studies of their use are small in number and they should be used with caution in patients with significant cardiac disease. The role of the newer agent modafanil is not yet established.

When cataracts become a problem they can be extracted with equally good results to senile cataracts. A careful examination should be made of the retina however to ensure that visual loss is not due to the rare pigmentary retinal change seen in DM1.

Anaesthetic management

The most important management issues are outlined in Table 4.10. Patients are particularly sensitive to

Table 4.10 Anaesthetic considerations in myotonic dystrophy

Pre-operative
- Tell patients always to remind doctors that they have myotonic dystrophy
- Patient should wear Medic-Alert or carry similar warning cards
- Preoperative ECG and respiratory assessment
- No "out of hospital" anaesthesia

Intra-operative
- Avoid thiopentone
- Avoid suxamethonium and long-acting neuromuscular blockers
- Monitor for arrythmias in theatre and post-operatively

Post-operative
- Beware post-operative respiratory depression or airway obstruction
- Use respiratory depressant analgesics with caution and at low doses

depolarizing muscle relaxants such as suxamethonium, which should be avoided. The use of thiopentone is also associated with prolonged respiratory depression and this agent is generally not recommended, especially in repeated doses. Finally patients with myotonic dystrophy require particularly close observation in the post-operative period for signs of respiratory depression, airways obstruction and arrhythmias. They are also at particular risk of post-operative chest infections.

Type 2 myotonic dystrophy or proximal myotonic myopathy (PROMM; DM2)

Proximal Myotonic Myopathy (PROMM) is a recently recognised autosomal dominant disorder characterised by proximal muscle weakness with atypical myotonia and pain. Most cases had initially been diagnosed as having atypical myotonic dystrophy. It is genetically separate from DM1, and the gene responsible localises to chromosome 3q21. It is allelic to the DM2, which is more similar to DM1 but not associated with the chromosome 19 triplet repeat mutation. DM2 appears commonest in families of Eastern European and, particularly, German origin. The genetic abnormality is an expansion mutation in a CCTG repeat sequence in the zinc finger protein 9 gene. The relationship between the size of the expansion and clinical severity is not yet clear. The prognosis is generally more benign than that of DM1.

The weakness in DM2 is proximal rather than distal, and the thigh muscles are particularly affected. The weakness in an individual may vary during the course of a day. One characteristic feature in patients is the complaint of pain in the muscles. Other points of difference from DM1 include muscle hypertrophy, asymmetry of myotonia and worsening of myotonia in some patients if the muscle is warmed.

Like DM1, DM2 is a multi-system disorder with cataracts which are indistinguishable from those in DM, cardiac arrhythmias, insulin resistance and CNS involvement shown by white matter changes on T_2-weighted MRI images. In contrast to DM1, higher mental function is rarely impaired but about a quarter of patients show an action tremor suggesting that the changes seen on neuroimaging may be relevant.

Diagnosis of DM2 currently is largely clinical. Investigations will show a normal or slightly elevated CK and myotonia on EMG testing. Genetic testing for the triplet repeat mutation in the myotonin protein kinase gene is negative. The myotonia cannot be reliably distinguished from that of DM1.

Congenital muscular dystrophy

The congenital muscular dystrophies (CMDs – Table 4.11) are a heterogeneous group of autosomal recessive disorders characterised by very early onset, generalised hypotonia, severe and early contractures and delayed motor milestones. The congenital myopathies (Chapter 11) are a different group, characterised by the presence of specific morphological abnormalities rather than the general dystrophic change seen in CMD.

The congenital muscular dystrophies share common pathological features with a "myopathic" pattern on muscle biopsy with variability in muscle fibre size and increased endomysial connective tissue. Necrotic and regenerative changes are seen only in the very early stages of the disorders. A distinctive feature (in biopsies from patients under 4 years old) is the presence of numerous muscle fibres with alkaline phosphatase staining, without evidence of inflammation or of other fibres degenerating (i.e. not showing acid phosphatase staining). One important point for classification is the presence or absence of merosin (laminin 2) since where staining is absent in muscle this correlates with more severe weakness and a failure to ever walk. About 50% of cases of CMD are merosin-deficient and form a heterogeneous group.

Merosin-deficient congenital muscular dystrophy

Merosin-deficient CMD is characterised by severe neonatal hypotonia, marked atrophy of limb and trunk muscles with weakness and multiple joint contractures which may be present before birth (arthrogryposis multiplex congenita). Kyphoscoliosis often also develops.

The pattern of weakness is predominantly proximal in the limbs, and weakness of the chest, face and neck are variable. In many cases there are problems with sucking and swallowing such that feeding is extremely problematic. Motor development is very much impaired but what motor skills are acquired tend not to be lost subsequently. The dystrophy thus appears to be relatively non-progressive.

Table 4.11   *Types of congenital muscular dystrophy (CMD)*

- CMD without symptomatic central nervous system involvement – classical CMD:
  - Merosin-negative
  - Merosin-positive
- CMD with other involvement:
  - Fukuyama CMD
  - Muscle-eye-brain (MEB) disease (Santavuori)
  - Walker-Warburg syndrome
  - CMD with familial junctional epidermolysis bullosa
  - CMD with early spine rigidity
  - CMD with mitochondrial structural abnormalities
  - CMD with respiratory failure and muscle hypertrophy

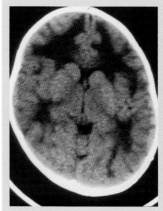

Figure 4.15
Magnetic resonance image changes in the brain of a patient with merosin-deficient congenital muscular dystrophy (T1-weighted). (Courtesy of Dr Stephanie A Robb.)

One major complication of the disease is respiratory involvement. Although of variable severity, respiratory muscle involvement is present from an early stage and attention to respiratory care is crucial from the time of diagnosis. Where there is kyphoscoliosis, there is a particular risk of retention of secretions and potentially life-threatening chest infections.

Intelligence is normal but white matter changes are consistently found on neuroimaging (Figure 4.15) and in some cases focal cortical dysplasias have been found. Up to 20% of patients have epilepsy.

Investigations reveal a raised CK (often markedly so early on in the disease) and a predominantly myopathic EMG, although slow motor nerve conduction may be found. The biopsy shows variation in fibre size within individual fascicles and rounding of fibres in cross section. Endomysial connective tissue is very prominent but fibre necrosis is rare and inflammation is not seen.

Merosin is the alternative name for α2 chain of laminin. Deletions, premature stop codons and occasional missense mutations all cause absence of merosin and CMD. It is coded on chromosome 6q2 and expressed in the basement membrane of muscle, skin, and both central and peripheral nervous tissue. It binds to β-dystroglycan, part of the dystrophin-associated protein complex, and to the basement membrane. Some cases of milder disease, with a later onset but still with changes on neuroimaging, are due to in-frame deletions which result in loss of the N-terminus of the protein.

Management of merosin-deficient CMD is supportive with particular attention paid to prevention and correction of contractures by passive stretching and splinting but avoiding surgery until weight bearing is achieved (if it is ever achieved). Parents must be taught about clearance of respiratory secretions and the importance of early treatment of chest infections.

Merosin-positive congenital muscular dystrophies

There are a number of other forms of CMD where merosin staining in muscle is normal. Some are a similar "pure" form of CMD, without significant involvement of other organ systems and in some of these patients α-actinin 3 is absent.

In addition there are other forms of CMD where there are associated CNS abnormalities. The best studied is Fukuyama-type CMD, a common form of muscular dystrophy in Japan but very rare in non-Japanese families. It is inherited as an autosomal recessive disorder and is associated with severe mental retardation and frequently with convulsions. Motor development is severely impaired with very few children ever able to stand or walk. Arthrogryposis is rare but contractures often develop in the first year of life. Facial weakness is marked, in contrast to many other forms of CMD. The gene responsible (at 9q31-q33) has been cloned and the protein product named fukutin. The protein has not been identified in normal muscle by immunocytochemistry, however, and it is though to be a secretory protein. Prognosis in Fukuyama CMD is poor with children rarely surviving far into their second decade.

Oculopharyngeal muscular dystrophy

This is a late-onset autosomal dominant condition characterised by a combination of ptosis, ophthalmoplegia and dysphagia. Typically onset is in the fourth to sixth decades of life with ptosis, which is often asymmetrical, with a progressive but usually incomplete ophthalmoplegia. Some homozygous cases have been described with an earlier onset. The ophthalmoplegia is rarely as marked as that seen in the chronic progressive external ophthalmoplegia of mitochondrial disease. Dysphagia and tongue weakness develop later. A large proportion of patients show some proximal limb weakness (most commonly in the lower limbs) if tested but it is only rarely striking and oculopharyngeal weakness dominates the clinical picture.

Diagnosis

Diagnosis is nowadays made by DNA analysis, so biopsy is not often required. Basic investigation reveals a normal or slightly elevated CK level. Raised levels usually occur where there is obvious involvement of limb musculature. The muscle biopsy appearances, where

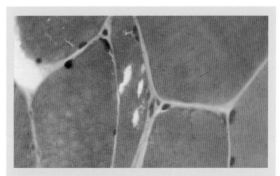

Figure 4.16 Oculopharyngeal muscular dystrophy. Rimmed vacuolar myopathy (Gomori trichrome)

performed, are those of a rimmed vacuolar myopathy with variability in fibre size and some angulated fibres (Figure 4.16). The rimmed vacuoles are not numerous, not membrane bound and may be seen associated with filaments similar to those in inclusion body myositis (IBM). Ultrastructurally, within the myocyte nucleus there are unique tubular filamentous inclusions (8.5 nm diameter) arranged in palisades or tangles. These inclusions are not seen in other cell types. In addition other 15nm diameter intranuclear inclusions similar to those seen in IBM may also be seen.

Genetics

OPMD may be inherited in an autosomal dominant or recessive fashion. The gene locus at chromosome 14q11.2-q13 codes for polyadenylate-binding protein-2 (PABP2) and the mutation lies within a guanine, cytosine, guanine (GCG) repeat encoding a polyalanine tract. In normal individuals there are 6 GCG repeats. In the recessive form of OPMD there is a homozygous expansion to 7 repeats, and in dominant OPMD a heterozygous expansion to either 8 or more commonly 9 repeats. Some cases with 7 repeats on one chromosome and 8 or 9 on the other have been described with a more severe phenotype. Unlike some of the other "triplet repeat" diseases such as myotonic dystrophy or Huntington's disease, the repeat expansion is stable with no increase in size between generations.

Management

The major treatment issues in OPMD relate to ptosis and dysphagia. Ptosis can be successfully treated either with props on spectacles or surgically with frontal suspension of the lids or resection of levator palpebrae. Dysphagia may respond to cricopharyngeal myotomy, although if there is evidence of coexisting gastro-oesophageal reflux or dysphonia the procedure is associated with unacceptable risks of aspiration. Under such circumstances, percutaneous gastrostomy should be considered.

Distal myopathies

The distal myopathies are a clinically and genetically heterogeneous group of disorders characterised by predominantly distal myopathic weakness. Obviously a major differential diagnosis is from neurogenic disorders, but a number of other muscle diseases classified separately also must be considered (Table 4.12). Inevitably, as with the LGMD group, advances in

Table 4.12 *Differential diagnosis of distal myopathy*

Myotonic dystrophy

Facioscapulohumeral dystrophy

Inclusion body myositis

Desmin storage diseases

Mitochondrial myopathy

Congenital myopathies

Glycogen storage disease (especially acid maltase deficiency)

Hereditary motor and sensory neuropathy (especially type II)

Distal spinal muscular atrophy

Davidenkow's syndrome

molecular genetics will allow a more rational and robust classification. It is possible now to classify the disorders by mode of inheritance (where this is clear), age of onset and the muscle group(s) that are first affected as well as by laboratory findings (Table 4.13). Even with this classification, the relation of hereditary inclusion body myopathy and oculopharyngodistal myopathy (Santoyoshi myopathy) to this group remains unclear.

In all forms of "pure distal myopathy" except Welander distal myopathy the onset is in the lower limbs. However there is spread to the upper limbs later in the disease in all forms but Udd myopathy (also known as Finnish tibial muscular dystrophy). The autosomal recessive (Miyoshi and Nonaka) distal myopathies may cause more generalised severe weakness and patients may become wheelchair bound. The Miyoshi form of distal myopathy in particular is associated with proximal weakness, especially of the glutei and biceps brachii and is allelic with type 2B LGMD. Although there have been occasional reports of involvement of cardiac muscle in patients with distal myopathies, it is not a consistent feature of any. In oculopharyngodistal myopathy (Santoyoshi myopathy) there is involvement of forearm muscles or the anterior tibial compartment followed by ptosis, ophthalmoplegia and dysphagia. Santoyoshi myopathy has been described in both autosomal recessive and dominant forms, but the relation of the dominant form to oculopharyngeal dystrophy is unclear.

Differentiation between the types of distal myopathy requires the integration of clinical information, CPK levels, EMG studies (especially to rule out myotonia or neuropathy) and muscle biopsy (Table 4.13). The muscle to be biopsied needs to be selected carefully. In early disease the changes may only be present in an affected muscle but in more severe cases there is a risk of obtaining only end-stage muscle. CT or MRI

Table 4.13 *Distal myopathies*

	Genetics	Muscle first affected	Age of onset	CPK	Biopsy RVs and TFIs	Fibre necrosis
Welander	AD 2p13	Hand/forearm – extensor	>40	N or ↑	+	+
Finnish type (Udd)*	AD 2p31	Leg – anterior	40–50	N or slight ↑	+	+
Markesberry–Griggs*	AD 2p31	Leg – anterior	25–50	2-5x ↑	+	–
Gowers–Laing	AD 14q11	Leg – anterior	4–25	3x ↑	–	+
Nonaka**	AR 9p1-q1	Leg – anterior	20–30	Up to 5x↑	+	–
Miyoshi = LGMD type 2b	AR 2p12-14 (Dysferlin)	Leg – posterior	15–30	10-100x↑	–	+

*These two conditions are almost certainly allelic

**Probably allelic with autosomal recessive hereditary inclusion body myopathy (IBM)

RVs = Rimmed vacuoles, TFIs = Tubulofilamentous inclusions

scanning can assist in choosing the best muscle for biopsy. Most of the genes responsible have been localised (Table 4.13) and it seems likely that Markesberry-Griggs and Udd myopathies are allelic and likewise Nonaka distal myopathy and a form of hereditary inclusion body myopathy with sparing of the quadriceps. Direct genetic testing is at present possible only for the dysferlin gene mutations causing Miyoshi type distal myopathy, however, and this is no simple task given the 55 exons to be tested.

Selected further reading

Barnes PRJ. Clinical and genetic aspects of myotonic dystrophy. *Brit J Hosp Med* 1993; 50: 2230.

Brais B, Bouchard JP, Xie YG et al. Short GCG expansions in the PABP2 gene cause oculopharyngeal muscular dystrophy. *Nat Genet* 1998; 18: 164–167.

Bushby KMD. Making sense of the limb-girdle muscular dystrophies. *Brain* 1999; 122: 1403–1420.

Bushby KMD, Gardner-Medwin D. The clinical, genetic and dystrophin characteristics of Becker muscular dystrophy. 1. Natural history. *J Neurol* 1992; 240: 998–1004

Emery AEH. *Duchenne Muscular Dystrophy* 2nd edn. Oxford: Oxford University Press, 1993.

Emery AEH. Emery-Dreifuss muscular dystrophy – a 40 year retrospective. *Neuromusc Dis* 2000; 10: 228–232.

Fitzsimons RB. Facioscapulohumeral muscular dystrophy. *Curr Opin Neurol* 1999; 12: 501–511.

Harper PS. *Myotonic Dystrophy* 3rd edn. London: WB Saunders, 2001.

Jöbsis GJ, de Visser M. Bethlem myopathy. In: Lane RJM (ed). *Handbook of Muscle Disease*. New York: Marcel Dekker, 1996.

Kakulas BA. The spectrum of dystrophinopathies. In: Lane RJM (ed). *Handbook of Muscle Disease*. New York: Marcel Dekker, 1996: 235–244.

Lim LE, Campbell KP. The sarcoglycan complex in limb-girdle muscular dystrophy. *Curr Opin Neurol* 1998; 11: 443–452.

Mastaglia FL, Laing NG. Distal myopathies: clinical and molecular diagnosis and classification. *J Neurol Neurosurg Psychiatry* 1999; 67: 703–709.

Matsumura K, Campbell KP. Dystrophin-glycoprotein complex: its role in the molecular pathogenesis of muscular dystrophies. *Muscle Nerve* 1994; 17: 2–15.

Ricker K. Myotonic dystrophy and proximal myotonic myopathy. *J Neurol* 1999; 246: 334–338.

Rowland LP, Hirano M, Di Mauro S, Schon EA. Oculopharyngeal muscular dystrophy, other ocular myopathies, and progressive external ophthalmoplegia. *Neuromusc Dis* 1997; 7(Suppl 1): 815–821.

Voit T. Congenital muscular dystrophies: 1997 update. *Brain & Development* 1998; 20: 65–74.

Wilhelmsen KC, Blake DM, Lynch T et al. Chromosome 12-linked autosomal dominant scapuloperoneal muscular dystrophy. *Ann Neurol* 1996; 39: 507–520.

chapter 5

Inflammatory myopathies

The inflammatory myopathies constitute a heterogeneous group of subacute, chronic, and rarely acute, acquired diseases of skeletal muscle which have in common the presence of moderate to severe muscle weakness and signs of endomysial inflammation. The diseases are clinically important because they represent the largest group of acquired and potentially treatable myopathies in children and adults.

A practical classification of all the inflammatory myopathies based on aetiology and pathogenesis is into: (a) idiopathic, probably autoimmune, which comprise the largest group, and (b) secondary, in association with other diseases, or infections. Based on distinct clinical, immunopathologic, histologic and prognostic criteria as well as different responses to therapies, the idiopathic, (autoimmune) IM are separated into 3 major and distinct subsets: polymyositis (PM), dermatomyositis (DM) and inclusion body myositis (IBM).

An autoimmune pathogenesis for PM, DM and IBM is strongly implicated based on their association with other putative or definite autoimmune diseases or viral infections, the evidence for a T-cell mediated myocytotoxicity or complement-mediated microangiopathy, and their varying response to immunotherapies. In IBM, the autoimmune features coexist with degenerative signs consisting of vacuolation, amyloid deposition and mitochondrial abnormalities. This chapter will review the main clinical and histological features of these diseases, their association with autoimmune conditions or viruses, and the underlying immunopathology. It also intends to provide a practical approach to immunotherapeutic interventions.

General clinical features

The incidence of polymyositis, dermatomyositis, and inclusion body myositis is approximately 1 in 100,000. Dermatomyositis affects both children and adults, and females more often than males, whereas polymyositis is seen after the second decade of life and very rarely in childhood. Inclusion-body myositis is three times more frequent in men than in women, is more common in Caucasians than in blacks, and is most likely to affect persons over the age of 50 years.

All three forms have in common a myopathy characterized by proximal and often symmetric muscle weakness that develops relatively slowly (weeks to months) and occasionally insidiously, as in inclusion body myositis, but rarely acutely. Patients usually report increasing difficulty with everyday tasks predominantly requiring the use of proximal muscles, such as getting up from a chair, climbing steps, stepping onto a curb, lifting objects, or combing their hair. Fine-motor movements that depend on the strength of distal muscles, such as buttoning a shirt, sewing, knitting, or writing, are affected only late in the course of dermatomyositis and polymyositis, but fairly early in inclusion-body myositis. Falling is common among patients with inclusion-body myositis because of early involvement of the quadriceps muscle and consequent buckling of the knees. Ocular muscles remain normal, even in advanced, untreated cases, and if these muscles are affected, the diagnosis of inflammatory myopathy should be in doubt. Facial muscle also remains normal except, rarely, in advanced cases. Mild facial muscle weakness however, is seen in up to 60% of patients with IBM. The pharyngeal and neck-flexor muscles are often involved, causing dysphagia or fatigue and weakness of neck flexion. In advanced cases and rarely in acute cases, respiratory muscles may also be affected. Severe weakness is almost always associated with muscular wasting. Sensation remains normal. The tendon reflexes are preserved but may be absent in severely weakened or atrophied muscles, especially in IBM where atrophy of the quadriceps and the distal muscles is common. Myalgia and muscle tenderness may occur in some patients, usually early in the disease, and more often in dermatomyositis than in polymyositis. Weakness in polymyositis and dermatomyositis progresses over a period of weeks or months, in contrast with the slower progression of muscular dystrophy, which is measured in years. Inclusion-body myositis may also progress slowly for years, and its clinical features may simulate those of limb-girdle muscular dystrophy.

Specific features

Dermatomyositis (DM)

DM occurs in both children and adults. It is a distinct clinical entity identified by a characteristic rash accompanying, or more often, preceding the muscle weakness. The skin manifestations include a heliotrope rash (blue-

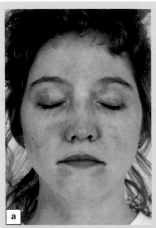
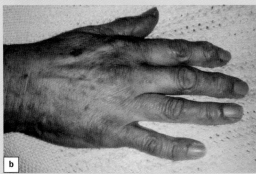
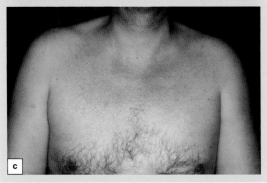

Figure 5.1 Clinical features of dermatomyositis. (a) Typical facial rash in dermatomyositis, including heliotrope discolouration of the eyelids. (b) Gottron's rash. (c) V shaped rash on the chest.

purple discoloration) on the upper eyelids with oedema (Figure 5.1a), a flat red rash on the face and upper truck, and erythema of the knuckles with a raised violaceous scaly eruption (Gottron rash – Figure 5.1b) that later results in scaling of the skin. The erythematous rash can also occur on other body surfaces, including the knees, elbows, malleoli, neck and anterior chest (often in a V sign – Figure 5.1c), or back and shoulders (shawl sign), and may be exacerbated after exposure to the sun. In some patients the rash is pruritic especially in the scalp, chest and back. Dilated capillary loops at the base of the fingernails are also characteristic of DM. The cuticles may be irregular, thickened, and distorted, and the lateral and palmar areas of the fingers may become rough and cracked, with irregular, "dirty" horizontal lines, resembling mechanic's hands. The degree of weakness can be mild, moderate or severe leading to quadraparesis. At times, the muscle strength appears normal, hence the tern "dermatomyositis sine myositis". When muscle biopsy is performed in such cases however, significant perivascular and perimysial inflammation is seen. In children, DM resembles the adult disease, except for more frequent extramuscular manifestations, as discussed later. A common early abnormality in children is "misery", defined as an irritable child that feels uncomfortable, has a red flush on the face, is fatigued, does not feel well to socialize and has a varying degree of proximal muscle weakness. A tiptoe gait due to flexion contracture of the ankles is also common.

DM usually occurs alone, but may overlap with systemic sclerosis, and mixed connective tissue disease. Fasciitis and skin changes similar to those found in DM have occurred in patients with the eosinophilia-myalgia syndrome associated with the ingestion of contaminated L-tryptophan.

Polymyositis (PM)

Patients with PM do not present with any unique clinical feature that heralds the diagnosis. Unlike in DM, in which the rash secures early recognition, the actual onset of PM cannot be easily determined. The patients present with subacute onset of proximal muscle weakness and myalgia that may exist for several months before they seek medical advise. In our judgement, the diagnosis of PM is one of exclusion. It is best diagnosed and defined as an inflammatory myopathy that develops subacutely, usually over weeks to months, progresses steadily and occurs in adults who do not have a rash, involvement of the extraocular and facial muscles (mild facial weakness is seen in IBM but not in PM), family history of a neuromuscular disease, history of exposure to myotoxic drugs or toxins, endocrinopathy, neurogenic disease, dystrophy, biochemical muscle disorder or inclusion-body myositis, as determined by muscle enzyme histochemistry and biochemistry.

Polymyositis can be viewed as a syndrome of diverse causes that may occur separately or in association with systemic autoimmune or connective tissue diseases and certain known viral or bacterial infections. Except for D-penicillamine and zidovudine, in which the myopathy is histologically characterized by endomysial inflammatory infiltrates similar to those seen in PM, myotoxic drugs do not cause PM. Instead, they elicit a toxic non-inflammatory myopathy that is histologically different from PM and does not require immunosuppressive therapy.

Inclusion-body myositis

IBM is the most common of the inflammatory myopathies. It affects men more often than women and it is most frequent above the age of 50 years. It is the most common acquired myopathy in men above 50 years old. Although IBM is commonly suspected when a patient

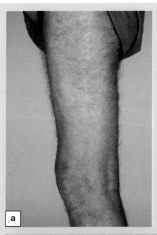
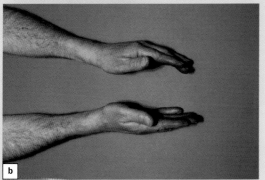

Figure 5.2
Inclusion body myositis. (a) Marked wasting of quadriceps. (b) Wasting of forearm flexor compartment.

with presumed polymyositis does not respond to therapy, involvement of distal muscles, especially foot extensors and deep finger flexors (Figure 5.2b), in almost all the cases, may be a clue to the early clinical diagnosis. Some patients present with falls because their knees collapse due to early weakness of the quadriceps muscles (Figure 5.2a). Others present with weakness in the small muscles of the hands especially finger flexors and complain of inability to hold certain objects such as golf clubs, to play the guitar, turn on keys or tie knots. The weakness and the accompanied atrophy can be asymmetric with selective involvement of the quadriceps, iliopsoas, triceps, biceps, and finger flexors in the forearm. Dysphagia is common, occurring in up to 60% of the patients, especially late in the disease. Because of the distal, and at times, asymmetric weakness and atrophy and the early loss of the patellar reflex owing to severe weakness of the quadriceps muscle, a lower motor neuron disease is often suspected, especially when the serum CK is not elevated. Sensory examination is generally normal except for a mildly diminished vibratory sensation at the ankles, presumably related to the patient's age. Contrary to early suggestions, the distal weakness does not represent neurogenic involvement but it is part of the distal myopathic process, as confirmed by macro EMG. In contrast to PM and DM in which facial muscles are spared, there is mild facial muscle weakness in 60% of IBM patients. The diagnosis is always made by the characteristic findings on the muscle biopsy, as discussed below.

Inclusion body myositis is associated with systemic autoimmune or connective tissue diseases in at least 20% of the cases. Hereditary cases, most often recessive and less frequently dominant, some with an associated leukoencephalopathy and others with sparing of the quadriceps, may be found. At present, the hereditary inclusion body myopathies include various ill-defined vacuolar, more commonly distal than proximal, myopathies with clinical profiles different from the one described above for sporadic IBM (s-IBM). Hereditary IBM with sparing of the quadriceps was first described in Iranian Jews but occurs also in other ethnic groups. Detailed descriptions and genetic data on h-IBM are not provided in this chapter because these diseases lack inflammation in their muscles and do not represent a true inflammatory myopathy. There is however a subset of patients with familial IBM that have the typical phenotype of sporadic IBM with histological and immunopathological features identical to the sporadic form.

Progression of IBM is slow but steady. The degree of disability in relation to the duration of the disease has not been systematically studied. Review of the course of 14 randomly chosen patients with symptoms for more than 5 years, revealed that 10 of them required a cane or support for ambulation by the fifth year after onset of disease while three of five patients with symptoms for 10 years or more were using wheelchairs for ambulation. Using quantitative muscle strength testing, we have found a 10% drop in muscle strength over a 1.5 year period. Recent data from 86 consecutive patients that we have studied, have shown that progression is faster when the disease begins later in life. The patients whose disease begins in their 50s may require the need for walking aids many years later compared to those patients whose disease begins in their 70s, presumably because of lesser reserves and diminished capacity for muscle regeneration in the older age groups.

Extramuscular manifestations

In addition to the primary disturbance of the skeletal muscles, extramuscular manifestations may be prominent in patients with inflammatory myopathies. These include: (a) dysphagia, most prominent in IBM and DM, due to involvement of the oropharyngeal striated muscles and distal oesophagus; (b) cardiac abnormalities consisting of atrioventricular conduction defects, tachyarrythmias, low ejection fraction and dilated cardiomyopathy either from the disease itself or from hypertension associated with long-term corticosteroid use; (c) pulmonary involvement, as the result of primary weakness of the thoracic muscles, drug-induced pneumonitis (e.g., from methotrexate), or interstitial lung disease. Interstitial lung disease may precede the myopathy or occur early in the disease and develops in up to 10% of patients with PM or DM, the majority of whom have anti-Jo-1 antibodies. Fatality related to adult respiratory distress syndrome has been noted in PM patients with anti-Jo-1 antibodies, emphasizing the diagnostic importance of these antibodies. Pulmonary capillaritis with varying degree of diffuse alveolar haemorrhage has been also described; (d) subcutaneous calcifications, sometimes extruding on the skin and causing ulcerations and infections, are found in some patients with DM, children more than adults; (e) gastrointestinal ulcerations seen more often in childhood DM, due to vasculitis and infection; (f) contractures of the joints especially in childhood DM; (g) general systemic disturbances, such as fever, malaise, weight loss, arthralgia, and Raynaud's phenomenon, when the inflammatory myopathy is associated with a connective tissue disorder; and (h) an increase incidence of malignancies in patients with DM, but not PM or IBM. Because tumours are usually uncovered not by a radiological blind search, but by abnormal findings on their medical history and physical examination, it is our practice to recommend a complete annual physical examination, with breast, pelvic and rectal examinations, urinalysis, complete blood-cell count, blood chemistry tests, and a chest X-ray film. Other investigations may be indicated by other co-existing clinical risk factors.

Diagnosis

The clinically suspected diagnosis of PM, DM, or IBM is established or confirmed by examining the serum muscle enzymes, the EMG findings and the muscle biopsy.

Serum muscle enzymes
The most sensitive enzyme is creatine kinase (CK), which in the presence of active disease can be elevated as much as 50 times the normal level. Although CK usually parallels the disease activity, it can be normal in active DM and rarely even in active PM. In IBM, CK is not usually elevated more than tenfold, and in some cases may be normal even from the beginning of the illness. CK may also be normal in patients with untreated, even active, childhood DM and in some patients with PM or DM associated with a connective tissue disease, reflecting the concentration of the pathologic process in the intramuscular vessels and the perimysium. Along with the CK, the serum aspartate transaminase (AST), serum alanine transaminase (ALT), lactate dehydrogenase (LDH) and aldolase may be elevated.

Electromyography
Needle electromyography shows myopathic potentials characterized by short-duration, low-amplitude polyphasic units on voluntary activation, and increased spontaneous activity with fibrillations, complex repetitive discharges, and positive sharp waves. This electromyographic pattern occurs in a variety of acute, toxic, and active myopathic processes and should not be considered diagnostic for the inflammatory myopathies. Mixed myopathic and apparently neurogenic potentials (polyphasic units of short and long duration) are more often seen in IBM but they can be seen in both PM and DM as a consequence of muscle fibre regeneration and

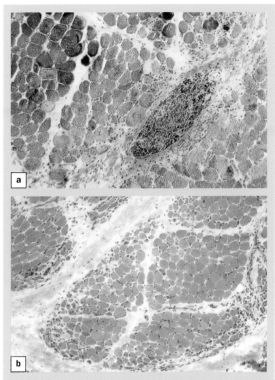

Figure 5.3 Muscle biopsy appearances in dermatomyositis. (a) Predominantly perivascular inflammatory infiltrate (Gomori trichrome stain). (b) Perifascicular atrophy. Note smaller fibres on the outside of the fascicle (H&E).

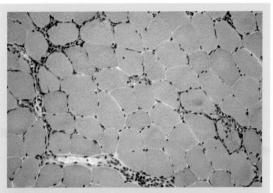

Figure 5.4 Muscle biopsy appearances in polymyositis. Note the inflammatory infiltrate between fibres and surrounding otherwise healthy fibres (H&E).

chronicity of the disease. Findings using macro-EMG have failed to show a neurogenic pattern of involvement in IBM patients. Electromyographic studies are generally useful for excluding neurogenic disorders and confirming either active or inactive myopathy.

Muscle biopsy

The muscle biopsy is the definitive test not only for establishing the diagnosis of DM, PM, or IBM, but also for excluding other neuromuscular diseases. Although the presence of inflammation is the histological hallmark for these disease, there are additional unique histological features characteristic for each group.

In DM the endomysial inflammation is predominantly perivascular or in the interfascicular septae and around rather than within the fascicles (Figure 5.3). The intramuscular blood vessels show endothelial hyperplasia with tubuloreticular profiles, fibrin thrombi, especially in children, and obliteration of capillaries. The muscle fibres undergo necrosis, degen-

eration and phagocytosis often in groups involving a portion of a muscle fascicle in a wedge-like shape, or at the periphery of the fascicle due to microinfarcts within the muscle. This results in perifascicular atrophy, characterized by two to ten layers of atrophic fibres at the periphery of the fascicles. The presence of perifascicular atrophy is diagnostic of DM, even in the absence of inflammation (Figure 5.3b).

In PM there is no perifascicular atrophy and the blood vessels are normal. The endomysial infiltrates are mostly within the fascicles surrounding individual, healthy, muscle fibres resulting in phagocytosis and necrosis (Figure 5.4). When the disease is chronic, the connective tissue is increased and often reacts positively with alkaline phosphatase.

The histological hallmarks of IBM are: (a) intense primary endomysial inflammation with T cells invading muscle fibres in a pattern identical to (but often more severe) the one seen in PM (Figure 5.5a); (b) basophilic granular deposits distributed around the edge of slit-like vacuoles (rimmed vacuoles) (Figure 5.5b); (c) loss of fibres (replaced by fat and connective tissue), and angulated or round fibres, scattered or in small groups; (d) eosinophilic cytoplasmic inclusions; (e) abnormal mitochondria manifested by the presence of ragged-red and cytochrome oxidase (COX)-negative fibres and supported by the frequent presence of mt-DNA deletions, seen in up to 75% of the patients; (f) tiny deposits of Congo-red or crystal violet-positive amyloid within or next to some vacuoles (Figure 5.5c). The amyloid, seen in approximately 80% of patients, immunoreacts with β-amyloid protein, the type of amyloid sequenced from the amyloid fibrils of the plaques from brains of patients with Alzheimer's disease;

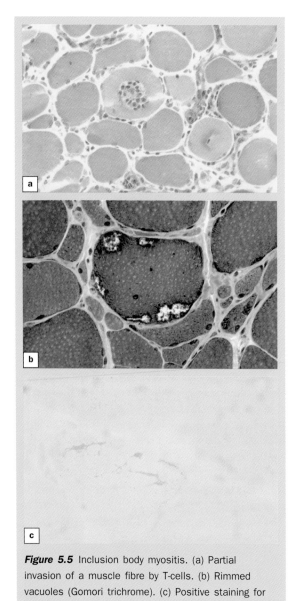

Figure 5.5 Inclusion body myositis. (a) Partial invasion of a muscle fibre by T-cells. (b) Rimmed vacuoles (Gomori trichrome). (c) Positive staining for amyloid (Congo Red).

(g) characteristic filamentous inclusions seen by electron microscopy in the cytoplasm or myonuclei, prominent in the vicinity of the rimmed vacuoles. Although demonstration of the filaments by electron microscopy was initially essential for the diagnosis of IBM, we do not feel that this is now necessary if all the characteristic light microscopic features including the amyloid deposits are fulfilled. Further, such filaments are not unique to IBM but they can be seen in other vacuolar myopathies. The cytoplasmic tubulofilaments within the vacuolated muscle fibres, as expected, immunoreact strongly with

amyloid-related proteins such as tau, ubiquitin, chymotrypsin and with prion protein.

Immune-mediated pathological mechanisms

Presence of autoantibodies

Various autoantibodies against nuclear (antinuclear antibodies) and cytoplasmic antigens are found in up to 20% of patients with inflammatory myopathies. The antibodies to cytoplasmic antigens are directed against cytoplasmic ribonucleoproteins which are involved in translation and protein synthesis. They include antibodies against various synthetases, translation factors, and proteins of the signal-recognition particles. The antibody directed against the histidyl-transfer RNA synthetase, called anti-Jo-1, accounts for 75% of all the anti-synthetases and it is clinically useful because up to 80% of patients with anti-Jo-1 antibodies have interstitial lung disease. In general, these antibodies may be non-muscle specific because they are directed against ubiquitous targets and they are almost always associated with interstitial lung disease even in patients who do not have active myositis. In addition, they are seen in all 3 subtypes (PM, DM and IBM), in spite of their clinical and immunopathological differences.

Immunopathology of dermatomyositis

The primary antigenic targets in DM are components of the vascular endothelium of the endomysial blood vessels and the capillaries. The earliest pathological alterations are changes in the endothelial cells consisting of pale and swollen cytoplasm with microvacuoles and undulating tubules in the smooth endoplasmic reticulum followed by obliteration, vascular necrosis and thrombi. Such alterations in the microvasculature occur early in the disease. The C5b-9 membranolytic attack complex (MAC), the lytic component of the complement pathway, is deposited on the capillaries before the onset of inflammatory or structural changes in the muscle fibres. Using an in vitro assay system that measures C3 consumption by sensitised erythrocytes on the basis of radiolabelled anti-C3 antibodies, it was further found that patients with active, but not chronic DM, have very high C3 uptake in their serum. MAC and the active fragments of the early complement components C3b and C4b were also found increased in the patients' serum using a radioimmunoassay.

The disease begins when putative antibodies directed against endothelial cells of the endomysium activate

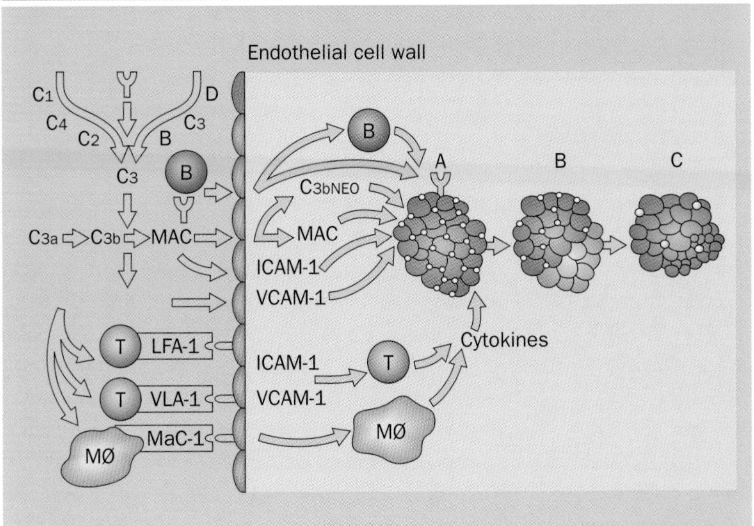

Figure 5.6 Immunopathology of polymyositis and inclusion body myositis.

complement C3 that forms C3b and C4b fragments and leads to formation and deposition of MAC on the endomysial microvasculature. The deposition of MAC leads, through osmotic lysis of the endothelial cells, to necrosis of the capillaries, perivascular inflammation, ischaemia and muscle fibre destruction, often resembling microinfarcts. The perifascicular atrophy often seen in more chronic stages is a reflection of the endofascicular hypoperfusion which is prominent distally. Finally there is marked reduction in the number of capillaries per each muscle fibre with dilatation of the remaining capillaries in an effort to compensate for the impaired perfusion. This process is diagrammatically depicted in Figure 5.6.

The putative anti-endothelial cell antibodies that fix complement can be detected by ELISA using human umbilical vein endothelial cells as antigen. However, characterization of the pathogenicity of these antibodies has not yet been performed. The activation of complement by the putative anti-endothelial cell antibodies is believed to be responsible for the induction of cytokines which, in turn, upregulate the expression of VCAM-I and ICAM-I on the endothelial cells and facilitate the exit of activated lymphoid cells to the perimysial and endomysial spaces (Figure 5.6).

Immunophenotypic analysis of the lymphocytic infiltrates in the muscle biopsies of patients with DM demonstrates that B cells and CD4$^+$ cells are the predominant cells in the perimysial and perivascular regions, supporting the view of a humoral mediated process, as described above.

Immunopathology of polymyositis and inclusion body myositis

Cytotoxic T cells

In PM and IBM, there is evidence not of microangiopathy and muscle ischaemia, as in DM, but of an antigen-directed cytotoxicity mediated by cytotoxic T cells. This conclusion is supported by the presence of CD8$^+$ cells, which along with macrophages initially surround healthy, but MHC-I-class expressing, non-necrotic muscle fibres that eventually invade and destroy them. These T-cells are activated, as evidenced by their expression of ICAM-I and MHC-I and II antigens on their surface, and exert a cytotoxic effect against muscle fibres as supported by the following:

(a) cell lines established from muscle biopsies of PM patients exert cytotoxicity to their autologous myotubes in vitro.
(b) by immunoelectronmicroscopy, CD8$^+$ cells and macrophages send spike-like processes into non-necrotic muscle fibres, which traverse the basal

lamina and focally displace or compress the muscle fibres.

(c) The cytotoxic autoinvasive CD8+ T cells contain perforin and granzyme granules which are directed towards the surface of the fibres and upon release they induce pores in the cell membrane and cell destruction. Efforts to document apoptotic cell death in these myofibres have repeatedly failed. The prevailing view at the moment is that destruction of the myofibre in PM and s-IBM is due to necrosis that takes place slowly but steadily.

(d) On the basis of T-cell receptor analysis, there is clonal expansion of T cells with restricted usage of TCR variable region of certain TCR gene families, notably Va1, Vb15 and Vb6, indicating that the T cell response is driven by a muscle-specific antigen. This is true not only for PM but also for s-IBM. In the latter, Vβ3, Vβ6 and Vβ5 gene families of the TCR of the autoinvasive CD8+ T cells were most frequently found, and when cloned and sequenced restriction in the amino acid sequence of the joining CD3 region was found.

(e) The cytotoxicity mediated by the CD8+ cells appears to be antigen-specific because, in addition to clonal expansion of certain TCR gene families described above, the T cells invade muscle fibres expressing MHC-I class antigen, a prerequisite for antigen recognition by the CD8+ cells. MHC-I class antigen is not present on normal muscle fibres but it is ubiquitously expressed on the sarcolemma of the muscle fibres in patients with PM and IBM. MHC-I expression is probably upregulated by cytokines secreted by activated T cells, macrophages or viruses (in a setting of a viral infection), as discussed later. Recent data indicate that the muscle fibres in PM and s-IBM express the BB1 marker of the antigen-presenting cells and their auto-invasive T cells express the CTLA-4 and CD28 counter-receptor. It appears therefore, that the muscle fibres are not only targets of cytotoxicity but they have also the potential to behave as antigen presenting cells. The nature of the antigenic peptides bound by the MHC-I for presentation to the CD8+ cells, remains still unknown. It is believed that such antigens are probably endogenous sarcolemmal or cytoplasmic self proteins synthesized within the muscle fibre. The possibility of being endogenous viral peptides appears unlikely because several laboratories have failed to amplify viruses within the muscle fibres not only in patients with PM triggered by a putative

viral infection, but also in patients with classic PM associated with HIV-1 or HTLV-1 infection.

(f) In 3 rare cases, γ/δ T cells or NK cells were the main participating cells in the myocytoxicity of PM and IBM.

(g) Expression of metalloproteinases MMP-2 and MMP-9. These zinc-dependent endopeptidases have been found upregulated on the MHC-I-expressing fibres and some CD8+ autoinvasive T cells. Because the muscle membrane contains extracellular matrix proteins such as collagen IV and fibronectin which are substrates for MMP-2 and MMP-9, these metalloproteinases may facilitate adhesion of T cells to the muscle and enhance cytotoxicity.

Cytokines and adhesion molecules

The T-cell derived cytokines (IL2, IL4, IL5 and TNF-γ), the macrophage-derived cytokines (IL1, IL6 and TNF-α), and cytokines that are either T-cell or macrophage-derived such as GM-CSF and TGF-β have been variably amplified with the reverse transcriptase-PCR method in the muscles of patients with PM, DM and IBM. Among the adhesion molecules and their receptors, ICAM-1, VCAM, ELAM, and their respective ligands, integrins β1 and β2, are also upregulated on the endothelial cells or the infiltrating T cells in patients with PM, DM and IBM and may facilitate the adhesion, penetration and exit of activated T cells through the endothelial cell wall. Collectively, a diagrammatic representation of the immunopathology of PM and s-IBM as shown in Figure 5.7.

Association with viral infections

Several viruses, including Coxsackie viruses, influenza, paramyxoviruses, CMV and EBV have been indirectly associated with chronic and acute myositis. A possible molecular mimicry phenomenon has been proposed with the Coxsackie viruses because of structural homology between the Jo-1, a histidyl-transfer RNA synthetase mentioned earlier, and the genomic RNA of an animal picornavirus, the encephalomyocarditis virus. Our very sensitive PCR studies however have repeatedly failed to confirm the presence of such viruses in these patients' muscle biopsies suggesting that it is unlikely, although not impossible, for these viruses to replicate in the muscles of patients with PM, DM and IBM.

The best evidence of a viral connection in PM and IBM is with retroviruses which have been associated with inflammatory myopathy in monkeys infected with the simian immunodeficiency virus, and in humans infected with HIV and HTLV-I. In HIV-positive patients, an

---

IMMUNOPATHOLOGICAL CHANGES IN DERMATOMYOSITIS

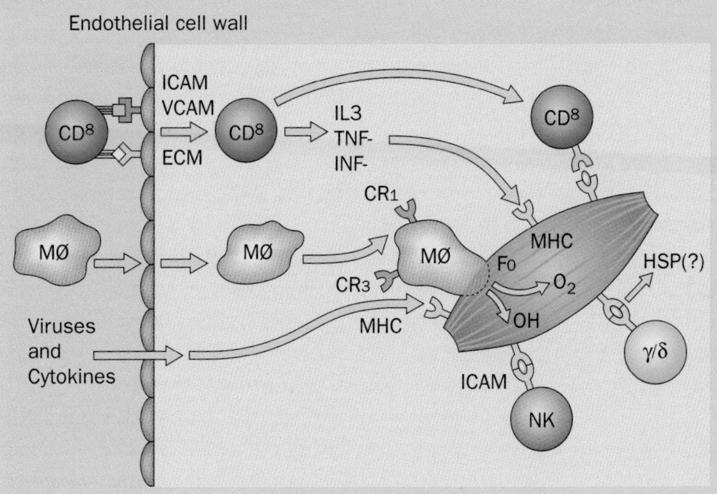

Figure 5.7 Immunopathological changes in dermatomyositis.

---

inflammatory myopathy (HIV-PM) can occur either as an isolated clinical phenomenon, being the first clinical indication of HIV infection, or concurrently with other manifestations of the acquired immune deficiency syndrome (AIDS). HIV seroconversion can also coincide with myoglobinuria and acute myalgia, suggesting that myotropism for HIV may be symptomatic early in the infection. In addition, HTLV-1 does not only cause a myeloneuropathy – referred to as tropical spastic paraparesis (TSP) – but also polymyositis, which may coexist with TSP or may be the only clinical manifestation of HTLV-1 infection. Of interest, IBM can also occur in a setting of HIV or HTLV-I infection. Using in situ hybridisation, Polymerase Chain Reaction, immunocytochemistry, and electron microscopy we could not detect viral antigens within the muscle fibres of these patients' muscle biopsies but only in occasional endomysial macrophages. We have interpreted these observations to suggest that in HIV- and HTLV-1 PM and IBM there is no evidence of persistent infection, of the muscle fibre with the virus or viral replication within the muscle. The predominant endomysial cell in HIV-1 and HTLV-1 PM and IBM are CD8+, non viral-specific, cytotoxic T cells which along with macrophages invade or surround MHC-I-antigen-expressing non-necrotic muscle fibres. Because this immunopathological pattern is identical to the one described earlier for retroviral-negative PM and IBM, we have proposed that a T-

cell-mediated and MHC-I-restricted cytotoxic process is a common pathogenetic mechanism in both retroviral negative and retroviral-positive PM and IBM, but in the latter viral-induced cytokines trigger the process.

Parasitic myositis

Several animal parasites, such as protozoa (*Toxoplasma* spp., *Trypanosoma* spp.), cestodes (cysticerci), and nematodes (trichinae), may produce a focal or diffuse inflammatory myopathy known as parasitic polymyositis. A suppurative myositis, known as tropical polymyositis or pyomyositis may be produced by *Staphylococcus aureus*, *Yersinia* spp., *Streptococci*, or other anaerobes. Pyomyositis, a previous rarity in the West, can now be seen in rare patients with acquired immunodeficiency syndrome (AIDS). Certain bacteria, such as *Borrelia burgdorferi* of Lyme disease and *Legionella pneumophila* of legionnaire's disease may infrequently be the cause of polymyositis.

The role of non-immune factors in s-inclusion body myositis

In IBM, the presence of amyloid-positive deposits within some of the vacuolated muscle fibres, the noted abnormalities in the nuclei, the presence of abnormal mitochondria and the relative resistance of the disease to immunosuppressive therapies, indicate that in this disease in addition to the autoimmune components mentioned earlier, there is also a degenerative process.

The amyloid in IBM is accompanied by all the other proteins associated with the β-amyloid of Alzheimer's disease, including β-APP, chymotrypsin, apoE, and phosphorylated tau. Whether these deposits are secondary and related to the chronicity of the disease or are a generated de novo and contribute to disease pathogenesis is unclear. The same can be said for the mitochondrial abnormalities and the mitochondrial DNA deletions which are observed in up to 70% of IBM muscles. Although such mitochondrial changes are more frequently seen in IBM than in normal aging, it is unclear if they are primary or secondary or if they are enhanced by the upregulated cytokines.

Treatment

Because the specific target antigens in DM, PM and IBM are unknown, the immunosuppressive therapies are not selectively targeting the autoreactive T cells or the complement-mediated process on the intramuscular blood vessels. Instead, they are inducing a non-selective immunosuppression or immunomodulation. Further, many of these therapies are empirical, and mostly uncontrolled.

The goal of therapy in inflammatory myopathies is to improve the function in activities of-daily-living as the result of improvement in muscle strength. Although when the strength improves, the serum CK falls concurrently, the reverse is not always true because most of the immunosuppressive therapies can result in decrease of serum muscle enzymes without necessarily improving muscle strength. Unfortunately, this has been misinterpreted as "chemical improvement", and has formed the basis for the common habit of "chasing" or "treating" the CK level instead of the muscle weakness, a practice that has led to a prolonged use of unnecessary immunosuppressive drugs and erroneous assessment of their efficacy. The prudence of discontinuing these drugs if, after an adequate trial, they have only led to a reduction in CK and not to an objective improvement in muscle strength must be emphasized.

The following agents are used in the treatment of PM and DM (see also Chapter 3).

Corticosteroids

Prednisolone is the first in line drug of this empirical treatment. Its action is unclear but it may exert a benefi-

cial effect by inhibiting recruitment and migration of lymphocytes to the areas of muscle inflammation and interfering with the production of lymphokines. Its effect on lymphokine IL_1 may be important because IL_1 is myotoxic and it is secreted by the activated macrophages that invade the muscle fibres. Corticosteroid-induced suppression of ICAM-I may also be relevant because downregulation of ICAM-I can prevent the trafficking of lymphocytes across the endothelial cell wall towards the muscle fibres.

Because the effectiveness and relative safety of prednisolone therapy will determine the future need for stronger immunosuppressive drugs, our preference has been to start with a high-dose prednisolone, 80–100 mg/day, from early in the disease. After an initial period of 3–4 weeks, prednisolone is tapered over a 10-week period to 80–100 mg in a single daily, alternate-day by gradually reducing the alternate "off day" dose by 10 mg per week, or faster if necessitated by side effects, though this carries a greater risk of breakthrough of disease. If there is evidence of efficacy, and no serious side effects, the dosage is then reduced gradually by 5–10 mg every 3–4 weeks until the lowest possible dose that controls the disease is reached. If by the time the dosage has been reduced to 80–100 mg every other day (approximately 14 weeks after initiating therapy), there is no objective benefit (defined as increased muscle strength) the patient may be considered unresponsive to prednisolone and tapering is accelerated while the next-in-line immunosuppressive drug is started.

Although almost all the patients with bone fide PM or DM respond to corticosteroids to some degree and for some period of time, a number of them fail to respond or become corticosteroids-resistant. The decision to start an immunosuppressive drug in PM or DM patients is based on the following factors:

(a) need for its "corticosteroids-sparing" effect, when in spite of corticosteroids responsiveness the patient has developed significant complications;
(b) attempts to lower a high-corticosteroid dosage have repeatedly resulted in a new relapse;
(c) adequate dose of prednisolone for at least a 2–3 month period has been ineffective;
(d) rapidly progressive disease with evolving severe weakness and respiratory failure.

The preference for selecting the next in line immunosuppressive therapy is, however, empirical. The choice is usually based on one's own prejudices, personal experience with each drug and assessment of the relative efficacy/safety ratio. The following immuno-suppressive agents are then used:

Azathioprine

This is a derivative of 6-mercaptopurine and it is given orally. Although lower doses (1.5–2 mg/kg/day) are commonly used, we prefer higher doses, up to 3 mg/kg/day for effective immunosuppression. This drug is well tolerated, has fewer side effects and, empirically, it appears to be as effective for long-term therapy as the other drugs.

Methotrexate

This is an antagonist of folate metabolism. Although its superiority to azathioprine has not been established, it has a faster action than the former. It can be given intravenously over 20–60 min at weekly doses of 0.4 mg/kg up to 0.8 mg/kg with sufficient fluids, or orally starting at 7.5 mg weekly for the first 3 weeks, increasing it gradually by 2.5 mg/week up to a total of 25 mg weekly. A relevant side effect is methotrexate-pneumonitis which can be difficult to distinguish from the interstitial lung disease of the primary myopathy, often associated with Jo-1 antibodies, as described above.

Cyclophosphamide

This alkylating agent is given intravenously or orally, at doses of 2–2.5 mg/kg/day. Cyclophosphamide has been of limited effectiveness in our hands but occasional promising results have been reported by others.

Chlorambucil

This is an antimetabolite that has been tried in some patients with variable results.

Ciclosporin

Although the toxicity of ciclosporin (mainly hypertension and impaired renal function) can now be reduced by measuring optimal trough serum levels (which vary between 100 to 250 ng/ml), its effectiveness in PM and DM is uncertain. A report that low-doses of ciclosporin could be of benefit in children with DM needs confirmation. The advantage of ciclosporin is that it acts faster than azathioprine or methotrexate and the results (positive or negative) may be apparent early.

Plasmapheresis

Plasmapheresis has not been shown to be helpful in a double-blind, placebo-controlled study.

Total lymphoid irradiation

Total lymphoid irradiation has been helpful in rare patients and may have long-lasting benefit. The long-term side effects of this treatment, however, should be seriously considered before deciding on this experimental and rather extreme approach. Total lymphoid irradiation has been ineffective in IBM.

Intravenous immunoglobulin

Intravenous immunoglobulin (IVIg) is a promising, but very expensive, therapy. In uncontrolled studies, IVIg was reported to be effective. In the first double-blind study conducted for DM, we have demonstrated that IVIg is effective in patients with refractory DM. Not only the strength improves but also the underlying immunopathology may resolve. The improvement begins after the first IVIg infusion but it is clearly evident by the second monthly infusion. The benefit is short-lived (not more than 8 weeks) requiring repeated infusions every 6–8 weeks to maintain improvement.

The mechanism of action of IVIg in DM may be by inhibiting the deposition of activated complement fragment on the capillaries, by suppressing cytokines especially ICAM-I, or by saturating Fc receptors and interfering with the action of macrophages.

A controlled double-blind study for PM is still underway although the drug has been effective is up to 80% of the patients in uncontrolled studies.

IVIg also exerted some benefit, although not statistically significant, in up to 30% of patients with IBM in an early controlled double-blind study. Although the improvement was not dramatic, it made a difference to these patients' life styles. However, a second study that investigated if IVIg in combination with prednisolone is better than prednisolone alone showed no benefit of IVIg.

Until further control drug trials are completed, the following step-by-step empirical approach for the treatment of PM, DM, is suggested:

Step 1: High-dose prednisolone;
Step 2: If the need for "corticosteroid-sparing" effect arises, try azathioprine, or methotrexate;
Step 3: If step 2 fails, try high-dose intravenous immunoglobulin;
Step 4: if step 3 fails, consider a trial, with guarded optimism, of one of the following agents, chosen according to the patient's age, degree of disability, tolerance, experience with the drug and the patient's general health: ciclosporin, chlorambucil, cyclophosphamide.

Selected further reading

Askanas V, Engel WK. Sporadic inclusion-body myositis and hereditary inclusion-body myopathies: current concepts of diagnosis and pathogenesis. *Curr Opin Rheumatol* 1998; 10: 530–542.

Askanas V, Serratrice G, Engel, WK (eds). *Inclusion Body Myositis and Myopathies*. Cambridge: Cambridge University Press, 1998.

Dalakas MC (ed.) *Polymyositis and Dermatomyositis*. Boston: Butterworths, 1988.

Dalakas MC. Polymyositis, dermatomyositis, and inclusion-body myositis. *N Engl J Med* 1991; 325: 1487–1498.

Dalakas MC. Retroviral myopathies. In: Engel AG, Franzini-Armstrong C (eds). *Myology*. New York: McGraw-Hill, 1994: 1419–1437.

Dalakas MC, Illa I, Dambrosia JM et al. A controlled trial of high-dose intravenous immunoglobulin infusions as treatment for dermatomyositis. *N Engl J Med* 1993; 329: 1993–2000.

Dalakas MC, Sekul EA, Cupler EJ, Sivakumar K. The efficacy of high dose intravenous immunoglobulin (iv Ig) in patients with inclusion-body myositis (IBM). *Neurology* 1997; 48: 712–716.

Engel AG, Hohlfeld R, Banker BQ. The polymyositis and dermatomyositis syndromes. In: Engel AG, Franzini-Armstrong C (eds). *Myology*. New York: McGraw-Hill, 1994: 1335–1383.

Griggs RC, Askanas V, DiMauro S, Engel AG, Karpati G, Mendell JR et al. Inclusion body myositis and myopathies. *Ann Neurol* 1995; 38: 705–713.

chapter 6

Muscle channelopathies

Membrane ion channels are essential for the proper functioning of excitable cells such as neurones and muscle. It is therefore of little surprise that disorders of ion channel function (channelopathies) are becoming increasingly recognised as an important cause of neurological disease. The first recognised neurological channelopathies were muscle diseases. A mild disturbance of ion channel function may result in muscle membrane depolarisation that leads to hyperexcitability and the symptom of myotonia. A more severe channel disorder may result in prolonged depolarisation leading to muscle membrane hypoexcitability and weakness such as that seen in periodic paralysis. A further muscle channelopathy to be discussed in this chapter is malignant hyperthermia syndrome.

The myotonias are divided into dystrophic and non-dystrophic myotonias. In the dystrophic myotonias, the myotonia may be an important diagnostic sign but the symptoms and signs are dominated by muscle atrophy with weakness and by a variety of multi-system features (see Chapter 4). The known genetic defect in the commonest of the dystrophic myotonias, myotonic dystrophy, does not directly involve a channel gene but it is possible that the myotonia is the result of some distant effect of the 19q trinucleotide expansion on a channel gene. In the non-dystrophic myotonias the myotonia is the prominent feature and is directly due to an ion channel gene mutation. Non-dystrophic myotonias are either sodium or chloride channel gene disorders (Table 6.1). Schwartz–Jampel syndrome is a severe infantile onset generalised myotonia associated with skeletal malformations and of variable aetiology.

In the past there was a confusing multiplicity of terms used to delineate different cases of periodic paralysis based upon the association of attacks with changes in serum potassium concentration or temperature, and the association with myotonia. Now we are able to define the main categories of periodic paralysis in genetic terms: hyperkalaemic periodic paralysis (with or without myotonia) is due to mutations in the same sodium channel gene as affected in sodium channel myotonias. Hypokalaemic periodic paralysis is due to defects in either a calcium channel or sodium channel gene (Table 6.1). Andersen's syndrome is a hereditary periodic paralysis associated with dysmorphic features and cardiac conduction abnormalities. Periodic paralysis can also occur as an acquired syndrome, secondary periodic paralysis, which needs to be distinguished from its hereditary, i.e. primary, counterparts.

Malignant hyperthermia is a genetic susceptibility to muscle hypermetabolism which is genetically heterogeneous. The majority seem to be associated with calcium channel gene mutations.

Table 6.1 *Muscle channelopathies*

Channel	Locus	Gene	Disease	No. of mutations
Sodium	17q23	SCN4A1	Paramyotonia congenita	10
			Hyperkalaemic periodic paralysis	4
			Potassium-aggravated myotonias	7
			Hypokalaemic periodic paralysis	2
Chloride	7q35	CLCN1	Thomsen's disease	10
			Becker's disease	30
Calcium	1q 31-32	DHPR	Hypokalaemic periodic paralysis	3
	1q 31-32	DHPR	Malignant hyperthermia	2
	19q 12–13.2	RYR	Malignant hyperthermia	>20

Myotonias

Clinical analysis of myotonia
Symptoms
Myotonia describes impaired muscle relaxation and while some sufferers may recognise that this is their problem their main complaint is usually of muscle stiffness. Pain is not a normal feature of myotonia per se unless the myotonia is unusually severe.

Relationship to exercise
Classically myotonia wears off with repeated contractions and this is known as the "warm up" phenomenon. In some potassium-aggravated myotonias the stiffness is most evident in the period of rest (for up to 40 minutes) following exercise and this stiffness can persist for up to 2 hours. In Thomsen's disease generalised myotonia may be particularly obvious when attempting exercise after rest. In extreme cases getting up from a chair provokes sudden generalised myotonia resulting in falls. Myotonia which worsens during exercise, sometimes to the point of immobility, is described as being "paradoxical" and is a feature of paramyotonia congenita.

Effect of temperature
All myotonia tends to worsen in the cold but the myotonia seen in paradoxical myotonia is particularly exacerbated by cold.

Variability
Generally the myotonia is a constant feature but in myotonia fluctuans, one of the potassium aggravated myotonias, there is a daily variation in the severity of the myotonia.

Distribution
Myotonia may be generalised as in the chloride channel myotonias or localised as in paramyotonia congenita where the face and arms are most affected. When generalised, myotonia can result in difficulties in chewing, problems with fine manipulative tasks and, when the legs are affected, falls. Facial involvement may lead to a complaint that the face feels like a rigid mask, the eyelids are hard to open and that a smile becomes fixed. Since facial involvement is particularly common in paramyotonia congenita which is cold sensitive these symptoms are most evident when a cold wind is blowing on the face.

Associated weakness
Weakness may be an associated feature of some myotonias. In paramyotonia congenita the there may be episodes of weakness precipitated by cold or occurring after prolonged exercise. Transient weakness is a feature of Becker's myotonia congenita and this is particularly evident when initiating exercise after a period of rest. Such transient weakness usually disappears within 20 to 60 seconds of repeated contractions but it can be generalised and disabling. Lack of appreciation of the transient nature of this weakness can lead to the erroneous impression of fixed weakness and hence a misdiagnosis of myotonic dystrophy. In contrast Thomsen's disease may be associated with increased muscle strength and some of these patients are successful in sports requiring strength without speed, such as some forms of weight lifting.

Signs
Grip myotonia
Myotonia may be elicited by asking the patient to make a tight fist and then open their clenched hand as quickly as possible – grip myotonia. The response to repeated gripping and relaxation will determine whether there is classical or paradoxical myotonia. In classical myotonia, particularly that seen in Thomsen's disease, there may be an initial worsening of grip myotonia with the first 3 to 4 contractions before the warm up phenomenon is seen.

Eyelid myotonia
Eyelid myotonia may be evident as slow opening of the screwed up eyelids and may also result in lid lag resembling that seen in thyroid disorders.

Percussion myotonia
Percussion of a myotonic muscle may initiate prolonged contraction sometimes with indentation of the muscle. Such percussion myotonia is typically elicited on percussion of the thenar eminence causing opposition of the thumb, but it can also be seen as wrist extension with slowed wrist drop after percussion of the forearm extensors. The napkin ring sign refers to the indentation of the protruding tongue caused by percussion against a sharp edge such as that of a tongue depressor. The hassle of eliciting the napkin sign means it is rarely worthwhile clinically.

Weakness
Episodic weakness occurring in paramyotonia congenita has the features of periodic paralysis (see below). Transient weakness is a particular feature of Becker's myotonia congenita and is best elicited by asking the patient to clench their fist tightly especially

after they have rested the hand for 5 to 10 minutes. Within seconds the grip becomes weak but it will recover after 20 to 60 seconds of repeated contractions.

Hypertrophy

Muscle hypertrophy is seen most commonly with the chloride channel myotonias (Thomsen's and Becker's diseases), and it may be more evident in the legs. In some cases calf hypertrophy may restrict ankle dorsiflexion. Hypertrophy of other muscles such as the neck may occur in the more severe forms of myotonia such as myotonia permanans and Schwarz-Jampel syndrome.

Sodium channel myotonias
Paramyotonia congenita

This disease is autosomal dominant, inherited with complete penetrance. Symptoms are usually present from birth and persist throughout life. The predominant symptom is that of paradoxical myotonia aggravated by cold temperatures. The myotonia particularly affects the face, neck and forearms. Typically on relief of the myotonia, either spontaneously or on warming, there is a variable degree of weakness which can persist for several hours. In a warm environment patients may have no symptoms at all. In some families with this disorder, there is a tendency for episodic weakness to occur independent of the myotonia. In such patients these attacks are precipitated by potassium ingestion, in much the same way as hyperkalaemic periodic paralysis. First attacks tend to appear in adolescence.

Potassium-aggravated myotonias

This is a group of recently classified myotonias, which have been shown to be due to mutations of the α1 subunit of the skeletal muscle sodium channel but which do not have the features of the other sodium channel disorders namely paramyotonia congenita and hyperkalaemic periodic paralysis. Before the advent of DNA based diagnosis many of these were diagnosed as myotonia congenita. They share the features of provocation by potassium load and of exacerbation of myotonia during a period of rest following exercise. The mildest phenotype is myotonia fluctuans in which the myotonia fluctuates on a daily basis being sometimes absent for days or weeks at a time. Acetazolamide-responsive myotonia is characterised by mild persistent myotonia with occasional painful muscle spasms worsened by the cold. As its name suggests it is responsive to acetazolamide. Myotonia permanens consists of unusually severe myotonia which can be painful and which can interfere with breathing. At least one such case was previously diagnosed as Schwartz-Jampel syndrome.

Chloride channel myotonias
Thomsen's disease

This is the less common, autosomal dominant form of chloride channel myotonia. It presents during the first decade of life with painless, generalised classical myotonia showing warm up phenomenon. It is associated with muscle hypertrophy but not with muscle weakness. Symptoms tend to progress until adolescence and thereafter remain constant throughout life.

Becker's disease

This autosomal recessive chloride channel myotonia tends to present later than Thomsen's disease, in the second decade, but presentation at 2 or 3 years of age has been seen. The myotonia is generalised and usually more severe than seen in Thomsen's disease. Muscle hypertrophy of legs and buttocks may occur. Becker's disease is associated with transient weakness not seen in Thomsen's disease and this can be disabling.

Schwarz–Jampel syndrome

This consists of continuous and severe myotonia usually beginning in infancy. The severity of the myotonia results in a typical facial appearance, laryngospasm and hypertrophy of the muscles in the neck, shoulders and thighs. The face is mask like with blepharospasm and puckering of the lips and chin often provoked by crying or excitement. Skeletal malformations, contractures and short stature may accompany this syndrome but only some cases have the chondrodysplastic features which give them the alternative name of chondrodysplastic myotonia. This syndrome has a heterogeneous pathophysiology as evidenced by the fact that the EMG characteristics of the myotonia can be variable, sometimes resembling neuromyotonia rather than myotonia. At least one case has been found to have a sodium channel abnormality.

Investigation

The serum CK is usually normal but if raised reflects the degree of muscle hypertrophy seen in some cases of chloride channel myotonia. Myotonia may be detected as spontaneous activity on EMG but in paramyotonia congenita cooling of the muscle may be required before it is apparent. There may be a decrement in the compound muscle action potential following exercise or 30Hz repetitive stimulation. This is particularly seen in cases of Becker's disease and may relate to the phenomenon of transient weakness seen in that condition.

Table 6.2 *Management of myotonia*

Avoid
- anticholinesterases
- succinylcholine
- potassium supplements in hyperkalaemic periodic paralysis

Anaesthesia
- D-tubocurare preferred
- uncertain association with malignant hyperthermia; dantrolene pre-treatment not necessary

Treatment of myotonia
- membrane stabilising drugs
  - procainamide 125–1000 mg/day
  - quinine 200–1200 mg/day
  - mexilitene 150–1000 mg/day
  - phenytoin 300 mg/day
- acetazolamide (in cases of sodium channel myotonia) 125–750 mg/day
- non-specific drugs (if ones above fail)
  - diazepam
  - verapamil

Table 6.3 *Differential diagnosis of periodic paralysis*

Single or first attack
- Metabolic
  - hypercalcaemia
  - hypocalcaemia
  - hypophosphataemia
  - hypomagnesaemia
- Rhabdomyolysis
- Guillain-Barré syndrome
- Acute poliomyelitis
- Myasthenic syndromes

Repeated attacks
- Secondary periodic paralysis
- Primary periodic paralysis
  - hypokalaemic periodic paralysis
  - hyperkalaemic periodic paralysis

Muscle biopsy is of limited value in cases of non-dystrophic myotonia. Genetic testing for common mutations may be available.

Management

This includes that avoidance of precipitating factors as well as pharmacological treatment for the myotonia, usually with membrane stabilising drugs (Chapter 3). Some of the sodium channel myotonias have a good but unexplained response to acetazolamide. Mexilitene has the advantage that it can treat not just the myotonia but also the weakness seen in Becker's disease or paramyotonia congenita (Table 6.2)

The periodic paralyses

Symptoms and signs

Weakness usually starts in proximal lower limb muscles and may then become generalised resulting in a flaccid tetraparesis. Ocular and respiratory muscles are usually not affected. The reflexes and the amplitude of the compound muscle action potential diminish in proportion to the weakness so that eventually the patient is areflexic and the EMG shows no compound motor action potentials at all. Attacks may be more readily provoked in the cold and with stress. Rest after a period of exercise is a common trigger. Thus attacks may develop during the night following a day of exercise and patients awake with weakness. Carbohydrate load is a precipitant in hypokalaemic periodic paralysis, while potassium ingestion is a precipitant for hyperkalaemic periodic paralysis. In younger subjects the only detectable interictal abnormality may be eyelid myotonia. Interictal fixed proximal weakness may be seen when attacks have been occurring for some years.

Differential diagnosis

Faced with a first attack of periodic paralysis, the differential diagnosis has to include other causes of a flaccid areflexic tetraparesis without sensory signs (Table 6.3). With repeated attacks most of these diagnoses fall by the wayside and the main diagnosis is between primary and secondary periodic paralysis and then between the two forms of primary periodic paralysis, including thyrotoxic periodic paralysis.

Primary versus secondary periodic paralysis

In many cases the history and associated features will point to the correct diagnosis. Secondary hypokalaemic periodic paralysis usually results from intracellular potassium depletion (typically to below a serum level of 2 mmol/l) from renal, endocrine, gastro-intestinal or drug-induced mechanisms (Table 6.4). Usually these underlying conditions are obvious but sometimes this is not the case and the recurrent episodes of transient weakness, can then be difficult to distinguish from

Table 6.4 *Causes of secondary periodic paralysis*

Endocrine
- Primary hyperaldosteronism (Conn's syndrome)
- Thyrotoxic periodic paralysis

Renal
- Juxtaglomerular apparatus hyperplasia (Barrett's syndrome)
- Renal tubular acidosis
- Fanconi syndrome
- Recovery from acute tubular acidosis

Gastro-intestinal
- Villous adenoma
- Gastrointestinal fistula
- Pancreatic non-insulin secreting tumours with diarrhoea
- Non-tropical sprue
- Laxative abuse

Drug induced
- Amphotericin B
- Liquorice
- Corticosteroids
- p-Aminosalicylic acid
- Carbenoxalone
- Potassium-depleting diuretics

primary hypokalaemic periodic paralysis. Late onset hypokalaemic periodic paralysis beyond 30 years of age should raise strong suspicions of secondary rather than primary periodic paralysis, including thyrotoxic period paralysis. Thyrotoxic periodic paralysis results from alteration of muscle membrane permeability and is commonest in Japanese, Chinese and other Asian populations but does occur in Caucasians. The clinical presentation is often indistinguishable from hypokalaemic periodic paralysis but with the additional, sometimes subtle, evidence of hyperthyroidism. Episodes of periodic paralysis may also precede the occurrence of obvious hypothyroidism.

Hyperkalaemic periodic paralysis

As with its allelic counterpart, paramyotonia congenita, hyperkalaemic periodic paralysis normally appears in infancy or early childhood with frequent episodes of paralysis which are generally brief and mild and last between 15 minutes to 4 hours. Attacks are typically triggered by potassium ingestion and they tend to occur at rest particularly if this follows exercise. The frequency of attacks may decline as the patient gets older. In some families with hyperkalaemic periodic paralysis, there is co-existent clinical myotonia which is usually mild while in others myotonia is only evident on EMG.

Hypokalaemic periodic paralysis

Primary hypokalaemic periodic paralysis is an autosomal dominant disorder but with variable penetrance in females; it thus appears to be more common in males. Attacks usually start by adolescence and invariably before the age of 30 years. The frequency of attacks is generally less than that seen in hyperkalaemic periodic paralysis and can vary from daily to only one or two in a lifetime. Attacks may be triggered by a carbohydrate meal and may be more likely to occur at times of stress. Typically attacks last between 1 to 4 hours but occasionally they can persist for up to 3 days. Fatalities are rare and usually result from injudicious treatment and hypokalaemia-induced cardiac dysrhythmias. Oliguria is typical during attacks and results from the intracellular sequestration of water.

Andersen's syndrome

This is an autosomal dominant condition, although sporadic cases have been reported. It consists of a triad of periodic paralysis, primary cardiac dysrhythmias (i.e. not related to serum potassium concentration) and dysmorphic features. The full triad is not always present. Some cases only ever have a single attack of periodic paralysis while others may have them every few weeks. They last several hours during which time the serum potassium concentration may show a variable response meaning that these attacks cannot be truly assigned to either the hyper- or hypo-kalaemic category. A whole range of cardiac rhythm abnormalities have been reported with the commonest being long QT syndrome. The dysmorphic features include hypertelorism, low set ears, broad nose and small mandible but the facial features are usually subtle. In some families with Andersen's syndrome mutations in the inward rectifying potassium channel gene KCNJ2 on chromosome 17q have been found.

Investigation of suspected periodic paralysis

Blood tests, ECG, and neurophysiology investigation are appropriate as detailed in Table 6.5. The short exercise test is a useful screening test for periodic paralysis (Table 6.6). In some cases provocative testing by way of hypokalaemic or hyperkalaemic challenge may be appropriate but needs close monitoring of electrolytes and ECG with facilities available to deal with any complications. It is therefore best left to experienced centres. It should not be done in those with a pre-existing cardiac dysrhythmia such as seen in Andersen's syndrome. Hypokalaemia is provoked by giving an oral glucose load which, if insufficient to

Table 6.5 *Investigation of periodic paralysis*

Blood tests		
Potassium	Serial assays may be required every 15–30 minutes to determine whether concentration is falling or rising during episode of paralysis	
Calcium	To exclude hypocalcaemia as a cause for muscle weakness	
Magnesium	To exclude hypomagnesaemia as a cause for muscle weakness	
Phosphate	To exclude hypophosphataemia as a cause for muscle weakness	
Creatine kinase	To exclude rhabdomyolysis as a cause for muscle weakness	
Thyroid function	To look for thyroid dysfunction associated with secondary hypokalaemic periodic paralysis	
Electrocardiogram	To look for evidence for hypo- or hyper-kalaemia and monitors for cardiac complications thereof	
Nerve conduction studies and repetitive stimulation	To exclude Guillain-Barré, botulism, myasthenia	
Electromyography	May detect myotonia in cases of hyperkalaemic periodic paralysis expect decrement in CMAP with periodic paralysis	
Muscle biopsy	May be abnormal; hypokalaemic periodic paralysis; large central vacuoles, necrotic fibres hyperkalaemic periodic paralysis; smaller vacuoles, tubular aggregates	

Table 6.6 *Short exercise test for periodic paralysis*

1. Measure baseline CMAP from abductor digiti minimi with stimulation of ulnar nerve
2. Ask patient to abduct little finger forcefully against resistance for 10 seconds
3. Repeat measurements of CMAP
4. Expect immediate decrement in CMAP amplitude with recovery within 5 minutes

CMAP = compound muscle action potential

provoke weakness, can be followed by an intravenous glucose load with insulin if required. Hyperkalaemia is induced by giving repeated doses of oral potassium chloride. In both types of challenge strength, reflexes and compound muscle action potentials are assessed at regular intervals.

Management

Preventative treatment includes the avoidance of precipitating factors as well as the use of prophylactic medication. The aim of such treatment is not just to prevent attacks but also to attempt to prevent the development of fixed inter-ictal weakness. Thus it should be considered even if attacks are mild. The management of acute attacks of periodic paralysis includes monitoring for complications with respiratory or cardiac support as required. While a variety of acute treatments can be used these are less necessary in the usually milder attacks seen in hyperkalaemic periodic paralysis. Attempts to correct the serum potassium should be guided by any cardiac complications. The potassium is rarely dangerously high in hyperkalaemic periodic paralysis. Low potassium concentrations are best treated with oral rather than intravenous potassium (Table 6.7). Treatment of thyroid disease is curative in cases of thyrotoxic hypokalaemic periodic paralysis.

Malignant hyperthermia

Malignant hyperthermia (MH) is a hereditary skeletal muscle disease characterised by a susceptibility to muscle hypercatabolism when exposed to anaesthetic agents. It has incidence of 1 in 12,000 anaesthetic incidents in children dropping to 1 in 50,000 anaesthetic events in adults. Males are more commonly affected than females. The peak incidence occurs at the age of 30 years following which the incidence declines to become very rare beyond the age of 75 years. Up to 1% of all children given halothane for anaesthesia seem to develop masseter muscle rigidity and it seems that up to half of these may be MH-susceptible. Although it is a genetically (and probably physiologically) diverse

Table 6.7 *Management of periodic paralysis*

Preventive measures
    In hypokalaemic PP – low carbohydrate diet; low sodium diet

Prophylactic treatment
    Acetazolamide
    Dichlorphenamide
    Thiazide diuretic in hyperkalaemic PP

Acute treatment
    Oral potassium if required in hypokalaemic PP
    Inhaled β-agonists (if no cardiac dysrhythmia)
    Avoid carbohydrate or potassium load which aggravate weakness in hyperkalaemic PP

Table 6.8 *Differential diagnosis of malignant hyperthermia*

Neuroleptic malignant syndrome
Acute dystonic reactions to drugs
Myotonic reaction to drugs
Lethal catatonia

Table 6.9 *Management of malignant hyperthermia*

Preventative
- Forewarn (e.g. MedicAlert bracelet)
- Avoid halothane
- Avoid suxamethonium

Supportive
- Cardiac support
- Respiratory support
- Renal support
- Treat hyperkalaemia
- Body cooling

Active treatment
- Intravenous dantrolene

condition and not all cases are proven to be due to channelopathy, the best understood form is due to a channelopathy and we therefore consider MH here.

Susceptible individuals rarely have any muscle symptoms except when exposed to a triggering event (although there may be an asymptomatic elevation of CK). This is often exposure to halothane general anaesthesia. The muscle relaxant succinylcholine is a milder trigger of attacks when used alone, but a more potent one when combined with halothane. The likelihood of triggering an attack with these agents is increased if the patient has been exercising vigorously beforehand or is under stress at the time of anaesthetic induction. Not every exposure triggers attacks, so patients may have had previous uneventful anaesthesia. Attacks frequently start with jaw spasm leading to generalised muscle spasm and rigidity. There may be associated hyperventilation, tachycardia, labile blood pressure and a mottled cyanotic skin rash. Within 15 minutes the body temperature may start to rise precipitously followed by metabolic and respiratory acidosis, hypoxaemia, generalised vasoconstriction and an increased cardiac output. End tidal Pco_2 usually rises before other parameters and before clinical signs (so that an appropriate monitor should always be used when anaesthetising a susceptible individual). The serum potassium may rise and the creatine kinase (CK) may rise 100 fold. Complications of myoglobinuria and disseminated intravascular coagulation may occur, either of which can lead to renal failure.

Differential diagnosis
These are listed in Table 6.8. Neuroleptic malignant syndrome can occur in response to dopamine blocking agents and typically occurs in psychiatric patients on neuroleptic drugs. Just as in malignant hyperthermia these patients can develop rigidity with hyperthermia and a raised creatine kinase. Generalised rigidity can also occur as a result of an acute dystonic reaction to neuroleptics or antiemetics. Patients with myotonia may develop rigidity with depolarising agents during anaesthetic induction.

Disease associations
As both central core disease (CCD) and malignant hyperthermia can result from mutations in the same ryanodine receptor *RYR* gene, it is unsurprising that CCD may present with malignant hyperthermia. Some of the clinical features of malignant hyperthermia may occur in a variety of other muscle diseases during general anaesthesia (see Chapter 3) but none appear to have a common genetic causation with malignant hyperthermia.

Management
Management of malignant hyperthermia (Table 6.9) begins with preventative measures, the most important of which is forewarning of possibly at-risk patients and advising them to carry appropriate documentation,

pendants or bracelets to let others know of the risk. Given such warning one can avoid the major precipitating agents of halothane and succinyl choline. It is safe to give such patients narcotics, barbiturates, benzodiazepines, nitrous oxide and depolarising muscle relaxants. Acute management consists of the removal of the triggering agents and the monitoring of cardiac renal and respiratory function so that appropriate supportive treatment can be given. Body cooling may be required in response to the hyperpyrexia which if allowed to continue aggravates the metabolic derangement. Dantrolene is the mainstay of treatment and given intravenously results in reversal of the abnormalities. Attention to these principles has resulted in a dramatic drop in mortality from 65% to 2%.

Screening

Evaluation of otherwise well patients thought to be at risk of developing malignant hyperthermia can be difficult. Only a few have a raised creatine kinase. The genetic heterogeneity and the fact that even the recognised point mutations only cover a small percentage of the patients at risk, limits the value of genetic testing.

A variety of in vivo tests have been purported to highlight at-risk individuals but these are not particularly reliable. The recognised screening test is the in vitro caffeine and halothane contracture test in which one looks for a lower than normal contractile threshold and exaggerated response to caffeine and/or halothane in freshly isolated muscle. This test is performed only in specialised centres, and even in these centres the overlap between normal and affected individuals is such that false positive tests are invariable. In pragmatic terms it may be best to treat someone as being "at risk" rather than trying exhaustive measures to exclude the possibility.

Pathophysiology and genetics of the channelopathies

Sodium channelopathies

The genetic basis of these sodium channel disorders is mutations in the *SCN4A* gene located on chromosome 17q23 and encoding for the α1 subunit of the skeletal muscle sodium channel (Figure 6.1). The mutations

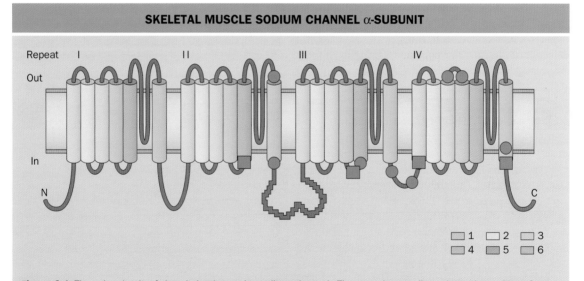

SKELETAL MUSCLE SODIUM CHANNEL α-SUBUNIT

Figure 6.1 The α1 subunit of the skeletal muscle sodium channel. The complete sodium channel consists of one α1 and one β subunit. Each α1 subunit, as shown here, consists of four identical domains labelled here as I to IV. Each domain contains six transmembrane segments labelled here 1 to 6. The transmembrane segments are linked by loops. Segment 4 (S4) acts as the voltage sensor controlling the opening or 'gating' of the channel. The cytoplasmic loop between segments 5 and 6 (the S5–S6 loop) of each domain lines the pores of the channel. The long cytoplasmic tail between domains III and IV occludes the pore by folding into it: the so-called 'hinge-lid'. The solid squares show the site of the four commonest mutations causing hyperkalaemic periodic paralysis, while the solid circles show the site of the known point mutations causing myotonia.

cause amino acid substitutions in sites likely to interfere with normal channel function such as the inactivation linker, the voltage sensor or the channel pore. Although some are associated with given phenotypes there are overlaps between the phenotypes (Table 6.1).

The mutant sodium channels display a reduction in fast inactivation of the sodium channel and some mutations also cause delay in slow inactivation of the channel. The muscle membrane contains a mixture of wild type and mutation containing channels. A mild defect of fast inactivation allows a small persistent sodium current which causes a mild depolarisation of the muscle membrane. This mild depolarisation triggers the re-opening of the fully recovered wild type normal sodium channels leading to a self sustained train of repetitive action potentials and delayed relaxation of the muscle i.e. myotonia. A more severe defect of sodium channel fast inactivation causes prolonged depolarisation of the membrane sufficient to inactivate wild type as well as mutant sodium channels making the membrane refractory to further stimuli and resulting in paralysis. Recovery from either the stiffness or the paralysis depends on restoration of the normal resting membrane potential by the sodium-potassium pumps.

Paradoxical myotonia with subsequent weakness occurs because exercise necessitates an increase in the rate of sodium channel openings to generate the required action potentials thus making the inactivation defect more obvious. The potassium sensitivity of these disorders is due to the fact that an elevation of the potassium level causes depolarisation of the membrane and increases the probability of sodium channel openings thus exposing the inactivation defect. The mechanism by which cold provokes symptoms in the sodium channel disorders remains unclear.

Chloride channelopathies

The over-excitability seen in the Thomsen and Becker myotonias is due to a reduced resting chloride conductance of the membrane. In normal muscle there is accumulation of potassium in the transverse tubules which could lead to depolarisation and hyper-excitability of the muscle were it not for the chloride current which balances it. When chloride conductance is impaired this potassium induced depolarisation gives rise to myotonia. This defect is associated with mutations in the chloride channel gene *CLCN1* on chromosome 7q32 (Figure 6.2). Dominant mutations are rare and some show a founder effect. Recessive mutations are much more common and may be homozygous or compound heterozygous. The genotype-phenotype correlations for these *CLCN1* mutations are incompletely understood. Generally dominant mutations result in greater reduction of the chloride conductance than do recessive mutations but the reduction in chloride conductance does not necessarily correlate with the severity of the myotonia. Some mutations can behave in both a dominant or recessive fashion. Perhaps these inconsistencies are explained

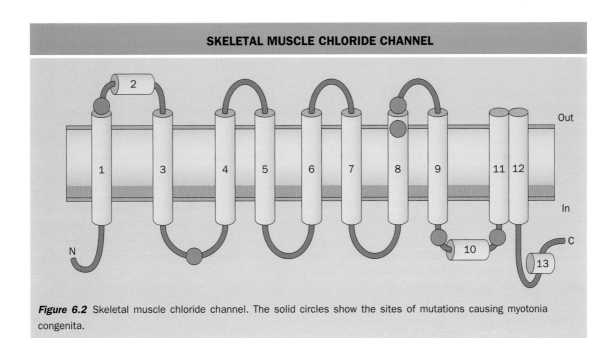

Figure 6.2 Skeletal muscle chloride channel. The solid circles show the sites of mutations causing myotonia congenita.

SKELETAL MUSCLE CALCIUM α1-SUBUNIT

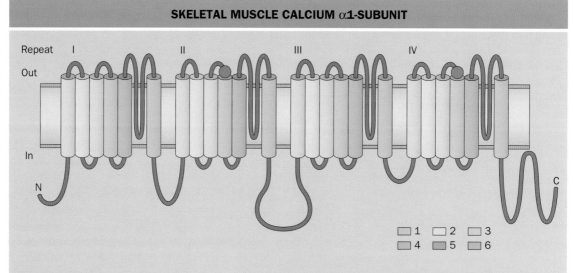

Figure 6.3 Skeletal muscle calcium channel α1-subunit. Note the similarities in structure with the α1 subunit of the sodium channel described in Figure 6.1. The solid circles show the sites of mutations causing hypokalaemic periodic paralysis.

by the effect of polymorphic variations elsewhere in the gene.

Calcium channelopathies

There are two major inter-related calcium channels in skeletal muscle: the dihydropyridine receptor and the ryanodine receptor which between them facilitate excitation-contraction coupling by releasing calcium from the muscle sarcoplasmic reticulum. The dihydropyridine receptor rather than being a channel per se acts as a voltage sensor for the ryanodine receptor which actually initiates the calcium release.

Three mutations in the *CACN1A3* gene on chromosome 1q31-q32 coding for the α1 subunit of dihydropyridine receptor (Figure 6.3) have been found in association with hypokalaemic periodic paralysis. There is no evidence of a founder effect and de novo mutations can occur. In hypokalaemic periodic paralysis there is an accumulation of intracellular potassium due to increased sensitivity to the potassium shifting action of insulin (independent of its glucopenic action). This may underlie the precipitation of attacks by carbohydrate load. The intracellular shift of potassium is accompanied by an influx of extracellular water causing the oliguria seen during attacks. However it is unclear

how this intracellular accumulation of potassium causes the sustained depolarisation seen in hypokalaemic periodic paralysis as normally intracellular potassium causes hyperpolarisation. Moreover, the role of the calcium channel in this process is still unclear.

Two to five percent of cases of malignant hyperthermia have mutations of the ryanodine receptor gene on chromosome 19q 13.2 (*RYR*). To date more than 20 point mutations in *RYR* have been described and all are located in the ligand-binding site for this receptor. Mutant channels show a heightened response of the channel to a variety of ligands with the channel being more easily activated and less readily inhibited. This impairment of channel function causes an increase in calcium level leading to continuous activation of the actin-myosin contraction apparatus and sustained muscle contraction. The continuous muscle activity results in the muscle rigidity, the muscle necrosis, the hyperpyrexia and the features of hypermetabolism.

In two families with malignant hyperthermia mutations were found in the same calcium channel gene as is implicated in hypokalaemic periodic paralysis. In other families linkage has also been found to chromosome 17q 1.2–24, which codes for the α subunit of the sodium channel, and to chromosome 7q and 3q.

Selected further reading

Engel AG, Franzini-Armstrong C (eds). *Myology* 2nd edn. New York: McGraw-Hill, 1994.

Fontaine B, Nicole S, Topaloglu H et al. Recessive Schwartz-Jampel syndrome (SJS): confirmation of linkage to chromosome 1p, evidence of genetic homogeneity and reduction of the SJS locus to a 3-cM interval. *Hum Genet* 1996; 98: 380-385

Griggs RC, Bender AN, Tawil R. A puzzling case of periodic paralysis. *Muscle Nerve* 1996; 19: 362-364.

Hanna MG, Stewart J, Schapira AH et al (1998). Salbutamol treatment in a patient with hyperkalaemic periodic paralysis due to a mutation in the skeletal muscle sodium channel gene (SCN4A). *J Neurol Neurosurg Psychiatry* 65: 248-250.

Lehmann-Horn F, Rudel R. Hereditary nondystrophic myotonias and periodic paralyses. *Curr Opin Neurol* 1995; 8: 402-410.

Lehmann-Horn F, Rudel R. Channelopathies: the nondystrophic myotonias and periodic paralyses. *Semin Ped Neurol* 1996; 3: 122-139.

Plaster NM, Tawil R, Tristani-Firouzi M et al. Mutations in Kir 2.1 cause the developmental and episodic electrical phenotypes of Andersen's syndrome. *Cell* 2001; 105: 511-519.

Ptacek LJ, Tawil R, Griggs RC et al. Sodium channel mutations in acetazolamide-responsive myotonia congenita, paramyotonia congenita, and hyperkalemic periodic paralysis. *Neurology* 1994; 44: 1500-1503.

Ricker K, Moxley RT, Heine R, Lehmann-Horn F. Myotonia fluctuans. A third type of muscle sodium channel disease. *Arch Neurol* 1994; 51:1095-1102.

Rose MR, Griggs RC (eds). *Channelopathies of the Nervous System*. Oxford: Butterworth Heinemann, 2001.

Sansone V, Griggs RC, Meola G S et al. Andersen's syndrome: a distinct periodic paralysis. *Ann Neurol* 1997; 42: 305-312.

Tawil R, Griggs RC, Rose MR. Channelopathies In: Pulst SM (ed). *Neurogenetics* (Contemporary Neurology Series) Philadelphia, USA: F.A. Davis Company, 2000: 45-60.

Tawil R, McDermott MP, Brown R, Jr. et al. Randomized trials of dichlorphenamide in the periodic paralyses. Working Group on Periodic Paralysis. *Ann Neurol* 2000; 47: 46-53.

Zhang J, George AL, Griggs RC et al. Mutations in the human skeletal muscle chloride channel gene (CLCN1) associated with dominant and recessive myotonia congenita. *Neurology* 1996; 47: 993-998.

Mitochondrial diseases of muscle

There are a huge number of biochemical process that take place within the mitochondria (Figure 7.1) which if abnormal can affect a variety of organ systems including skeletal muscle. This chapter will concentrate on those defects which particularly affect skeletal muscle, specifically defects of oxidative phosphorylation and of β-oxidation. The former group are the traditional "mitochondrial myopathies" characterised by the proliferation of mitochondria which is best seen as ragged red fibres in Gomori trichrome stained muscle biopsy. Even though β-oxidation is a mitochondrial process the defects of this system do not result in ragged red fibres

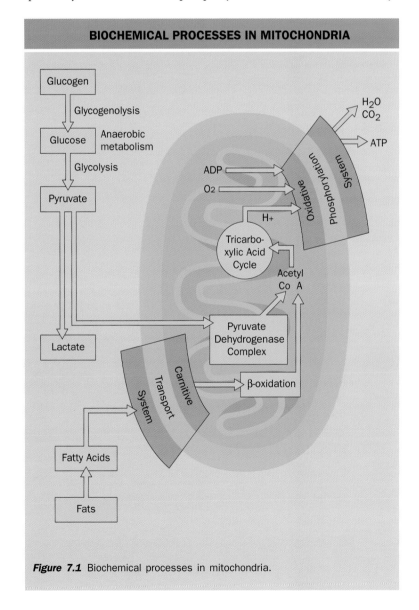

Figure 7.1 Biochemical processes in mitochondria.

and so are not usually included as "mitochondrial myopathies". Both mitochondrial respiratory chain and β-oxidation defects can be associated with multi-system neurological and non-neurological involvement and these features will also be mentioned.

Defects of oxidative phosphorylation – mitochondrial myopathies

Introduction
Basic biochemistry
The oxidative phosphorylation system is located in the inner membrane of the mitochondrion, is responsible for the oxidation of substrates derived from glycolysis and β-oxidation and uses the energy so derived to

regenerate ATP from ADP. It consists of the four multimeric protein subunits of the respiratory chain (Complexes I, II, III and IV) which pass electrons down an energy gradient while protons are extruded across the mitochondrial inner membrane. This creates a "proton motive force" which is discharged through Complex V resulting in the phosphorylation of ADP to ATP (Figure 7.2). The oxidative phosphorylation system is unique in that 13 of the 80 or more protein subunits which make up the respiratory chain complexes are encoded for by mitochondrial DNA (mtDNA) (Table 7.1).

Properties of mtDNA
Mitochondrial DNA has a number of special properties which have a bearing on disease expression (Table 7.2) It is a small genome of 16.5 kB which nevertheless packs

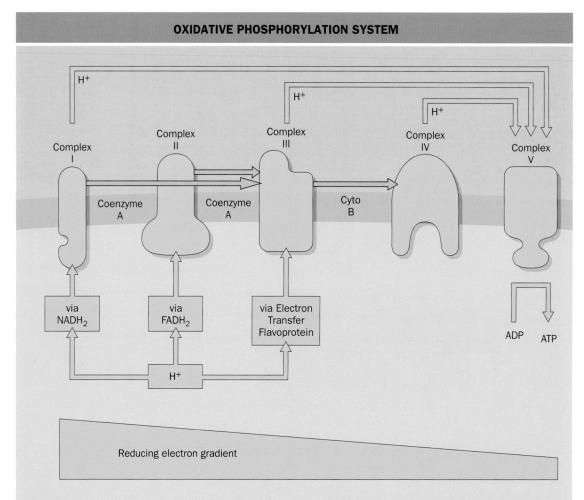

Figure 7.2 The oxidative phosphorylation system. NADH = nicotinamide adenine dinucleotide; FADH2 = flavin adenine dinucleotide; CoA = Coenzyme A; Cyt B = Cytochrome B; H+ = protons.

Table 7.1 Genomic origin of oxidative phosphorylation system

Complex No.	Name	Polypeptides	
		Total	mtDNA
I	NADH-ubiquinone reductase	26 approx	7
II	Succinate-ubiquinone reductase	4	0
III	Ubiquinol-cytochrome C reductase	11	1
IV	Cytochrome C oxidase	13	3
V	ATP synthase		2

Table 7.2 Properties of mtDNA

Property	Disease consequence
Maternally inherited	Mitochondrial myopathies may be maternally inherited
Multiple copy number	mtDNA mutations may be heteroplasmic
No introns	Mutations more likely to be deleterious
Lacks full repair mechanisms	High spontaneous mutation rate
Is only semi-autonomous	There are other mechanisms for the aetiology of mitochondrial myopathies other than through primary defects of mtDNA

in not only the 13 protein coding genes but also genes for 2 rRNAs and 22 tRNAs (Figure 7.3). This efficiency is possible because of the absence of non-coding DNA sequences (introns), the use of smaller tRNAs than seen in nuclear DNA and by the "multi-tasking" of some genes which not only code for their respective proteins but also function as stop codons or punctuation between flanking gene sequences. However these properties mean that mutations of mtDNA are more likely to be deleterious and may affect mtDNA function in more

than one way. MtDNA exists in the biochemically hostile environment of the mitochondrial matrix exposed to free radicals and this, together with its paucity of repair mechanisms, accounts for its high

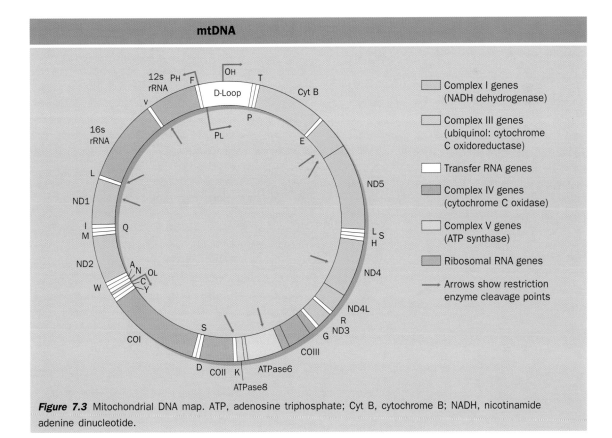

Figure 7.3 Mitochondrial DNA map. ATP, adenosine triphosphate; Cyt B, cytochrome B; NADH, nicotinamide adenine dinucleotide.

spontaneous mutation rate. Each cell has multiple mitochondria each of which has between 8–10 copies of mtDNA (i.e. a mtDNA copy number of 8–10) not all of which may be affected by a given mtDNA mutation. These mutations are therefore described as heteroplasmic and may be quantified as the percentage of the total mtDNA pool affected by a given mutation. The percentage heteroplasmy for a given mutation may vary from one individual to another and from tissue to tissue within a given individual. Although mtDNA is autonomous so far as translation is concerned replication and transcription of mtDNA remains controlled by the nuclear genome. mtDNA is almost exclusively maternally inherited, so this pattern of inheritance may be a distinctive feature of some mitochondrial myopathies.

Biosynthesis of mitochondrial proteins

Since only a small proportion of mitochondrial respiratory chain proteins are mtDNA-encoded, the majority of the proteins which are nuclear DNA encoded (and thus synthesised in the cytosol) need to be imported to their final destination within the mitochondria in order to allow final assembly of a functional oxidative phosphorylation system. This highly specific and targeted import machinery is controlled by the nuclear genome.

Possible aetiologies for mitochondrial disease

The biosynthesis of the oxidative phosphorylation system just described allows the postulation of a number of mechanisms which could give rise to a defect of the oxidative phosphorylation system (Table 7.3). The literature contains examples of each of these mechanisms giving rise to mitochondrial disease. Mitochondrial myopathies can therefore be inherited or acquired. The pattern of inheritance can be autosomal, either dominant or recessive, or maternal. Spontaneous mtDNA mutations can also occur leading to sporadic cases.

Table 7.3 *Possible aetiologies for mitochondrial disease*

- Defects of the nuclear genome:
  - affecting nuclear encoded mitochondrial protein subunits
  - regulating mitochondrial genome function
  - regulating transport of cytoplasmic proteins into the mitochondria
- Defects of the mitochondrial genome affecting mitochondrial protein synthesis
- Defects of both genomes (bigenomic defects)
- Acquired defects of mitochondrial function

Factors influencing mitochondrial disease expression

The clinical expression of a mitochondrial defect depends upon the severity of the defect in terms of its effect on ATP production and upon the energy requirements of the tissue concerned.

The severity of the defect of respiratory chain function depends on the percentage heteroplasmy for a given mtDNA mutation which may vary from tissue to tissue. This variation in percentage heteroplasmy is most marked for single length deletions and less so for tRNA point mutations. In rapidly dividing tissues the mutation may be selected out. A dramatic example of this was a infant with Pearson's syndrome in which the haematological and hepatic features improved while the muscle features became more prominent and a Kearns-Sayre phenotype emerged. In post-mitotic tissue such as CNS and muscle the percentage heteroplasmy cannot decrease.

An equivalent impairment of ATP production may have little effect on skin as compared with its effect on tissues with higher energy demand such as kidney, heart, skeletal muscle or the central nervous system. Mitochondrial function also declines with age and this may alter the balance between ATP production and demand, leading to the worsening of existing symptoms or the emergence of new or additional symptoms. A precarious balance between ATP production and demand in a given tissue under basal conditions may become symptomatic under conditions of increased energy demand. For example muscle weakness may not be apparent at rest but appear during exertion thus accounting for the common feature of exertional fatigue in mitochondrial myopathy. Similarly CNS symptoms such as stroke-like events and encephalopathy may be triggered by the increased energy demands of an intercurrent illness.

MtDNA mutations and genotype-phenotype correlations

A number of different types of mtDNA mutations have been reported. Point mutations and single length deletions are primary mtDNA defects. Depletion of mtDNA and multiple length mtDNA deletions are secondary mtDNA defects resulting from a nuclear DNA defect that disrupts mtDNA replication. The mtDNA point mutations are maternally inherited while the single length deletions are usually sporadic and secondary mtDNA defects are inherited in an autosomal fashion. There is an ever expanding number of mtDNA mutations being described but some are more common than others (Table 7.4). A comprehensive and frequently updated list of the reported mtDNA

Table 7.4 *mtDNA mutations and abnormalities*

(Examples only given, for a comprehensive and updated list see http://www.gen.emory.edu/mitomap.html)

- Single deletions
  - common deletion 4977 bp long
- Multiple deletions
  - with common origin
  - with multiple origins
- Duplications of mtDNA
- Depletions of mtDNA
- Point mutations
  - of tRNA genes
    - tRNA leu 3243 MELAS or CPEO
    - tRNA leu 3271 MELAS
    - tRNA lys 8344 MERRF
    - tRNA lys 8356 MERRF
  - of protein coding genes
    - ND4 11778 LHON
    - ND1 4160 LHON
    - ND1 3460 LHON
    - A6 8993 NARP

mutations is available at http://www.gen.emory.edu/mitomap.html.

MtDNA point mutations may affect protein coding, tRNA, or rRNA genes. Deletions invariably affect both protein coding and tRNA genes. It seems that mutations affecting tRNA genes or mtDNA copy number are associated with mitochondrial proliferation which results in ragged red fibres seen on muscle biopsies of affected individuals. By contrast mutations of protein coding genes such as seen in Leber's Hereditary Optic Neuropathy (LHON) and in NARP (Neurogenic weakness, Ataxia, Retinitis Pigmentosa) do not seem to be associated with ragged red fibres

The relationship between specific mtDNA defects and the precise biochemical defect of the oxidative phosphorylation systems is poor. This may be in part due to the technical difficulties of biochemical analysis of respiratory chain function. Although some mtDNA mutations are associated with particular clinical phenotypes, such associations are not invariable or exclusive.

Clinical features

Myopathy

This may be the sole feature of the disease. In some the myopathy is not a presenting feature but is found on examination. The onset of muscle symptoms is usually in childhood or adolescence, but neonatal presentation, and late onset, in the fifth decade, have been described. The commonest distribution of weakness is of a proximal type with arms being more affected, however a facioscapulohumeral pattern may occur. The muscle weakness is usually mild and rarely results in loss of walking ability. Those who do lose walking ability usually have additional CNS features as the main cause. Myopathy is often associated with external ophthalmoplegia and in some cases pigmentary retinopathy is also present. Most of those presenting with muscle weakness do not develop CNS disease but those that do usually do so within 5 years. A positive family history is found in 50% of cases with isolated muscle weakness. Fatigable weakness is a common feature and this can be disabling. There may be exercise-induced cramps with or without myoglobinuria. Patients with muscle weakness have some degree of lactic acidaemia which increases on exercise. Some cases have episodic exacerbations of their muscle weakness, sometimes associated with headaches, nausea and vomiting with severe metabolic acidosis documented in a few. Precipitants for such attacks include intercurrent infection, alcohol and unaccustomed exertion.

Chronic progressive external ophthalmoplegia/ Kearns-Sayre syndrome

Chronic progressive external ophthalmoplegia (CPEO) is a very common manifestation of mitochondrial myopathy. Because it is insidious in onset patients may not appreciate its presence. There is usually impairment of eye movements in all directions of gaze but only rarely a complaint of diplopia. Accompanying ptosis may be asymmetrical or, rarely, unilateral. Frequent associations with CPEO include limb weakness and fatigue, cerebellar ataxia, short stature, delayed sexual maturation and other endocrine abnormalities, sensorineural deafness, myopathy, cardiac conduction defects, raised CSF protein and cranial or peripheral neuropathies. Pigmentary retinopathy is a common accompaniment and is usually of the salt and pepper type, although the more classic bone spicule pattern has also been seen. Visual failure and peripheral field constriction is not usually seen with the salt and pepper type pigmentary retinopathy but occurs more often with the classical form. The Kearns-Sayre syndrome forms a subset of those with CPEO. It is defined by the presence of three obligatory features; onset before 20 years old; ptosis and ophthalmoplegia; and pigmentary retinopathy with one of three other features: heart block, CSF protein greater than 100 mg/dl, or

Table 7.5 *Diagnostic criteria for Kearns-Sayre syndrome*

- Onset before 20 years of age of:
  - Ptosis with ophthalmoplegia
  - Pigmentary retinopathy
  - And one out of: cardiac conduction block; cerebellar ataxia; CSF protein >100 mg/dl

cerebellar ataxia (Table 7.5). Most of the CPEO group of mitochondrial myopathies represent sporadic cases although some familial cases have been described.

Single length mtDNA deletions are the commonest genetic basis for CPEO group especially in those with no CNS involvement and those with the Kearns-Sayre syndrome. However CPEO can also be associated with multiple mtDNA deletions and with mtDNA tRNA point mutations. Those patients having CPEO without CNS involvement usually have little if any disability.

Zidovudine myopathy

Zidovudine is an inhibitor of mtDNA polymerase γ and so can cause depletion of mtDNA with a consequent myopathy. The myopathy usually occurs in those having long-term zidovudine treatment and is a painful

Table 7.6 *Mitochondrial CNS syndromes*

Syndrome	Features	Notes
MERRF (Myoclonic Epilepsy with Ragged Red Fibres)	Myoclonic epilepsy, cerebellar ataxia, dementia, sensorineural deafness while less common are optic atrophy and a sensory peripheral axonopathy	
MELAS (mitochondrial Myopathy, Encephalopathy, Lactic Acidosis and Stroke-like episodes)	Stroke-like events are often preceded by migraine-like headache, nausea and vomiting	Distinguished from MERRF by lack of myoclonus, optic atrophy and peripheral neuropathy
Leigh syndrome	Affecting mainly infants and children; delayed milestones, dementia, seizures, cerebellar ataxia, nystagmus, optic atrophy, ptosis, ophthalmoplegia, deafness, spasticity, hypotonia, weakness, and anorexia with vomiting. Cardiac and renal complications of hypertrophic cardiomyopathy and Fanconi syndrome	Initially defined as a pathological entity characterised by a spongy necrosis of the CNS, with vascular proliferation and glial reaction
Alpers' syndrome	Developmental delay failure to thrive in infancy, intractable seizures, liver failure	
NARP (Neurogenic weakness, Ataxia and Retinitis Pigmentosa)	Retinitis pigmentosa, ataxia, dementia, seizures, proximal muscle weakness and sensory neuropathy	Maternally inherited, no ragged red fibres
MNGIE (Myo-Neuro-Gastro-Intestinal Encephalopathy)	Ophthalmoplegia, gastric and intestinal dysfunction and peripheral and autonomic neuropathy	
Infantile lactic acidaemias/ encephalopathies	Severe neonatal lactic acidaemia with respiratory embarrassment, feeding difficulties, failure to thrive, severe hypotonic weakness, mental impairment, seizures with renal, hepatic and cardiac involvement	
Multiple symmetrical lipomatoses	Multiple symmetrical lipomatoses and peripheral neuropathy with variable manifestations of deafness, myopathy, cerebellar and pyramidal features and seizures	
Pearson's syndrome	Usually fatal, neonatal pancreatic and hepatic dysfunction, pancytopenia and lactic acidosis	
Leber's Hereditary Optic Neuropathy (LHON)	Sub-acute, usually bilateral and sequential, progressive optic nerve degeneration	Maternally inherited, marked male preponderance, no ragged red fibres

proximal wasting myopathy with either a normal or only modestly raised creatine kinase. It usually improves following withdrawal of the drug. It may be difficult to differentiate zidovudine-induced myopathy from HIV related inflammatory myopathy. Muscle biopsies show inflammatory infiltrates with ragged red fibres and cytochrome oxidase negative fibres.

Cardiomyopathy

In a few families a cardiomyopathy usually with cardiomegaly and hypertrophy has been described. More commonly cardiac involvement is confined to varying degrees of conduction block and this is mostly seen in the CPEO group.

Neuropathy

This is a common but usually asymptomatic manifestation of mitochondrial disease. When symptoms do occur they usually consist of distal sensory loss, with motor symptoms being uncommon (although motor signs may be found). Nerve conduction studies usually show evidence of an axonopathy. More prominent neurogenic weakness is a feature of the NARP syndrome (Table 7.6).

Central nervous system

Encephalomyopathy and its associated symptoms usually appear in childhood or early adulthood although presentation at either extreme of life have been described. A major feature of this group is the occurrence of episodic headaches and vomiting, stroke-like events and seizures with dementia. Others have combinations of myoclonic epilepsy, ataxia, dementia and sensorineural deafness. These two presentations have been highlighted as specific syndromes in adults namely MERRF and MELAS (Table 7.6). Myopathy is usually mild in these cases and there may be neurophysiological evidence of muscle involvement in cases without clinically detectable weakness or fatigability. Extra-pyramidal features including dystonia and choreo-athetoid movements have been described. Widespread multiple necrotic foci, haemorrhage and spongioform degeneration of the brain are seen at post mortem. The ophthalmoplegia, retinopathy and cardiac conduction block characteristic of KSS are not generally seen in this group. The main features of the MERRF and MELAS syndrome as well as of other mitochondrial CNS syndromes are shown in Table 7.6. In reality many cases show overlap between the clinical features of these syndromes and the syndromes are not clearly defined in genetic terms either.

Table 7.7 *Differential diagnosis of mitochondrial muscle weakness*

With ophthalmoplegia	Myasthenic syndromes
	Oculopharyngeal muscular dystrophy
	Thyroid ophthalmopathy
With fatigue	Myasthenic syndromes
With neuropathy	Inclusion body myositis
	FSH dystrophy ("neurogenic" muscle biopsy)
	HIV myopathy with neuropathy
With CNS features	Myotonic dystrophy
	Duchenne muscular dystrophy
	Congenital myopathy with merosin deficiency

Non-neurological

Most non-neurological manifestations of mitochondrial disease are rare. Short stature and diabetes mellitus are relatively common. Other endocrine abnormalities can include hypothyroidism and growth hormone deficiency. Bone marrow failure can occur as in Pearson's disease and renal tubular defects may lead to a Fanconi's syndrome. Gastrointestinal symptoms of pseudo-obstruction and vomiting can occur with encephalopathy and these are also a feature of MNGIE (see Table 7.6).

Differential diagnosis

Each of the myriad features of mitochondrial disease has a differential diagnosis of its own. However often it is the combination of multi-system neurological and non-neurological manifestations which lead to a diagnosis of mitochondrial myopathy. In some cases mitochondrial disease remains the most likely diagnosis even in the absence of definitive proof. Table 7.7 summarises the additional features which may occur with mitochondrial myopathy and the differential diagnosis for each.

Investigations
Initial investigations

Routine haematological and biochemical investigations are usually normal. Exceptions to this would be the sideroblastic anaemia or pancytopenia seen in Pearson's syndrome or the biochemical abnormalities which can result from renal involvement causing a Fanconi's syndrome. Creatine kinase (CK) is usually normal even in those with prominent muscle involvement. Perhaps the most useful biochemical screen is the lactate concentration. Resting, fasting levels of lactate may be raised in serum, or in the case of disease confined to the CNS, in cerebrospinal fluid. CSF protein may be raised and this is one of the diagnostic criteria for Kearns-Sayre syndrome. An ECG may show cardiac conduction defects.

Exercise testing

Sometimes resting serum lactate is normal but carefully graded aerobic exercise may show a exaggerated rise and slow recovery of the lactate levels. The test should be performed on a rested and fasted individual. Blood samples are taken at rest and then immediately after 15 minutes of exercise and then 15 minutes later. The aim of the test is to stress oxidative phosphorylation capacity (i.e. mitochondrial function), while not overwhelming it, otherwise there will be a physiological switch to anaerobic metabolism which produces lactate anyway. The bicycle resistance is therefore continuously adjusted so as to ensure a constant sub-anaerobic workrate this being calculated from the subject's gender, age and weight. An example of the results obtained in a normal individual and one with mitochondrial myopathy are shown in Figure 7.4.

Neurophysiology

Electromyography may show myopathic features even in cases with apparently exclusive CNS involvement, but these features are not specific for mitochondrial disease. Similarly EEG may show non-specific

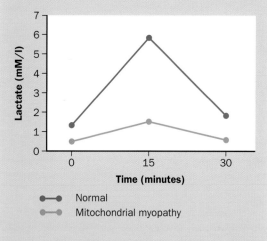

SUBANAEROBIC THRESHOLD EXERCISE TEST

Normal
Mitochondrial myopathy

Figure 7.4 Example of sub-anaerobic threshold bicycle exercise test result.

evidence of brain dysfunction as well as evidence of myoclonic and, or, generalised epileptiform activity. Nerve conduction studies may show evidence of a subclinical peripheral axonopathy which is said to be more often seen in MERRF. Subclinical hearing loss or retinal pathology may be disclosed by audiometry, and electro-retinograms respectively.

Imaging studies

Both computerised tomography (CT) and magnetic resonance imaging (MRI) may be abnormal in cases with CNS disease. Multiple low density CT, or high signal MRI lesions may be seen anywhere in the cerebral hemispheres or posterior fossa. There is a predilection, particularly in Leigh's disease, for the basal ganglia, where there may also be calcification. Sub-cortical white matter lesions may be seen. Wedge shaped lesions resembling vascular infarction may be seen especially in the MELAS syndrome. These are characteristically seen at the occipito-temporal junction thus resembling vascular watershed infarcts. Less specific findings of cerebral and, or, cerebellar atrophy may occur.

Functional studies

[31]Phosphorus nuclear magnetic resonance (^{31}P NMR) spectroscopy (see Chapter 2) performed on exercising muscle can show patterns of abnormality which are specific for respiratory chain impairment as opposed to other defects of muscle energy production. There is a low resting phosphocreatine (PCr) to inorganic phosphate (Pi) ratio which falls more rapidly on exercise. Despite the excess of lactic acid the rise in proton concentration is buffered by the consumption of protons which accompanies PCr breakdown. Thus there is only a small drop, and often a slight rise, in intracellular pH. On cessation of exercise, the pH recovers quickly, while recovery of PCr is delayed due to slow ATP synthesis. ^{31}P NMR spectroscopy of the brain has also revealed a defect of oxidative phosphorylation in one patient with mitochondrial encephalopathy. Positron emission tomography (PET) has shown, in three cases with known respiratory chain dysfunction, evidence for reduced cerebral oxygen consumption with glucose metabolism continuing, presumably anaerobically. This is consistent with impairment of oxidative phosphorylation.

Muscle biopsy

Histocytochemistry

The modified Gomori trichrome stain shows phospholipid as red and thus highlights the proliferation of mitochondria characteristic of these diseases. The red granular staining may be confined to the periphery of the fibres but may also be seen within the intermyofibrilar network with disruption of the fibrils giving rise to the ragged red fibre appearance. The intra-mitochondrial enzyme, succinate dehydrogenase (part of Complex II) may show a similar pattern of intense staining and may be more sensitive. There may also be excessive deposits of glycogen or lipid occurring as a secondary phenomenon and shown by the periodic acid Schiff (PAS), or Sudan black stains respectively. Stains for cytochrome oxidase activity can show negative staining fibres particularly in the CPEO group where they may be more numerous than ragged red fibres (Figures 7.5 and 7.6).

There is no correlation between the severity of the disease and the frequency of ragged red fibres. In some cases mitochondrial disease may exist without ragged red fibres but with cytochrome oxidase negative fibres. Conversely the presence of a few ragged red fibres does not necessarily imply a mitochondrial disease, particularly in the elderly. It is possible to have mitochondrial disease without ragged red fibres if the defect is confined to a mtDNA protein coding gene as in Leber's hereditary optic neuropathy and NARP.

Electron-microscopy

As well as being increased in numbers, mitochondria may show a variety of structural abnormalities which can be observed on electron-microscopy. The mitochondria can be greatly enlarged, have unusual arrangements of cristae, and contain abnormal inclusions. Cristae can be branched, concentric, peripherally located, or transverse within elongated mitochondria. Mitochondria may appear empty, vacuolated, or show granules which are similar to those seen in normal mitochondria, but larger and more prominent. Much bigger osmiophilic bodies may be present. Large regular rectangular structures may be seen either within the cristae or the intermembranous space. These paracrystaline inclusions may occupy part or the whole width of the mitochondria or may be present in small groups of four parallel stacked lines within a common outer membrane; the so-called parking lot inclusions. All these morphological abnormalities appear to be non-specific in that they do not indicate any precise biochemical defect. (Figure 7.7)

Biochemistry

Mitochondrial enzyme analyses can be performed using spectrophotometry on whole muscle homogenate and

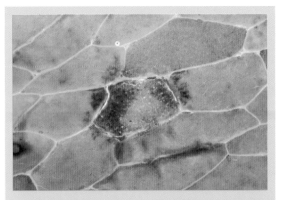

Figure 7.5 Muscle biopsy showing ragged red fibres.

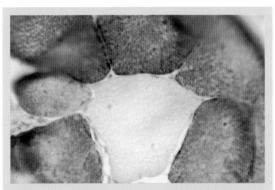

Figure 7.6 Muscle biopsy showing cytochrome oxidase negative fibres.

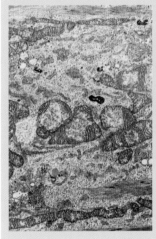

Figure 7.7 Electron micrograph of mitochondrial abnormalities.

results expressed as enzyme activities per g of citrate synthetase activity in order to correct for mitochondrial content. A much larger muscle sample is required to obtain intact mitochondria suitable for oxygen

Table 7.8 *Classification of polarographic defects of respiratory chain*

	Oxygen utilisation with		
	NAD-linked substrates interacting with complex I	Succinate interacting with complex III	Ascorbate + TMPD interacting with complex IV
No defect	Normal	Normal	Normal
Complex I deficiency	Decreased	Normal	Normal
Complex I-III deficiency	Decreased	Decreased	Normal
Complex I-IV deficiency	Decreased	Decreased	Decreased

electrode studies. In this technique samples of mitochondria are incubated with various substrates, in the presence of limiting amounts of ADP and the consumption of oxygen monitored polarographically. The different substrates feed electrons into the respiratory chain at different points, and this knowledge allows deduction of the site(s) of the defect of the respiratory chain. The results can be classified as shown in Table 7.8. The cytochromes can be assayed using room temperature or low temperature spectroscopy.

Molecular biology

Detection of deletions of mtDNA is most readily accomplished by digesting the mtDNA with an endonuclease which cuts the circular genome at a single site thereby linearising it. Where a deletion is present Southern blotting will then reveal two bands, the higher molecular weight wild type mtDNA, and a smaller molecular weight mutant mtDNA (Figure 7.8). Such analysis is generally done on total DNA extracted from muscle with radiolabelled mtDNA as the probe, without the need to separate out mtDNA. The Southern blot technique may not detect deletions in blood mtDNA and is usually performed on muscle DNA. Although deletion detection can also be achieved by selective amplification across the break point using polymerase chain reaction (PCR) this can be difficult to apply to blood DNA samples as non-selective amplification of nuclear DNA may give confusing results.

Point mutations of mtDNA may result in the loss or gain of a restriction site. PCR can be used to amplify the region of interest, and the PCR product digested with an appropriate endonuclease. Restriction site gain or loss can be detected following agarose gel electrophoresis visualisation of the digest under UV light following ethidium bromide staining. Point mutations are more readily detectable in blood DNA samples.

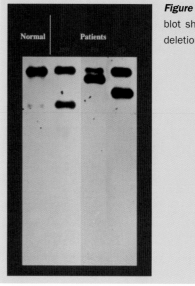

Figure 7.8 Southern blot showing mtDNA deletions.

Management of myopathy
General

Patients should be advised to avoid excessive exercise and alcohol which are recognised triggers for episodes of decompensation and lactic acidosis. With occasional exceptions patients with muscle weakness due to mitochondrial myopathy do not develop early respiratory weakness. However in parallel with advanced limb weakness respiratory failure can occur and may require supportive management (see Chapter 3 for details). The commonest cardiac feature is conduction block and regular monitoring for this particularly in those with CPEO may be life saving as the timely insertion of a cardiac pacemaker may prevent sudden death from dysrhythmia.

Ptosis

If ptosis intrudes on vision then treatment can be offered. Ptosis occurring without significant facial weakness may be amenable to surgery involving eyelid slings. Surgery requires a high level of expertise in order to prevent exposure conjunctivitis. However such surgery may become ineffective if and when facial weakness progresses. Ptosis in association with facial weakness may be successfully managed by the use of ptosis props on spectacles or else of special contact lenses that incorporate a shelf on which the eyelids can rest.

Biochemical treatment

Specific biochemical treatment is unsatisfactory. Several agents such as ubiquinol, carnitine, riboflavin, thiamine, succinate, ascorbate and menadione have been tried in an attempt to surmount the biochemical block in the mitochondrial respiratory chain but none are of proven effectiveness. In many cases there are multiple defects of respiratory chain function including downstream defects for which there are no available treatments. Corticosteroids have been of apparent benefit in some cases of mitochondrial encephalopathy.

Genetic counselling

The accuracy of genetic counselling is greatly enhanced when the specific gene defect is known. Even so predicting the onset or severity of the disease in asymptomatic but affected family members is difficult due to variability of phenotypic expression. Prenatal testing has been performed but the relationship between the degree of heteroplasmy in placenta for a given mtDNA mutation and eventual disease expression may be poor. Where there is no detectable mtDNA deletion and no mode of inheritance discernable the empirical figures suggest a recurrence rate of around 1–2% for the offspring of males and 10–20% for the offspring of females. For maternally inherited mtDNA mutations there may be the option of ovum donation.

Defects of β-oxidation

Introduction
Basic biochemistry

Long chain fatty acids are transported through the impermeable mitochondrial inner membrane using an active transport system that requires carnitine as a carrier with two carnitine palmitoyl transferases (CPT 1 and 2) and a carnitine-acylcarnitine transferase. CPT 1 is located on the outer mitochondrial membrane while CPT 2 and carnitine-acyl-carnitine transferase are embedded in the inner membrane. Subsequent β-oxidation involves the repetitive operation of a series of four enzymes each cycle of which sequentially cleaves off two carbon atoms as acetyl CoA. Eventually the fatty acyl CoA containing n carbon atoms is completely oxidised to $n/2$ acetyl CoA molecules. These acetyl CoA molecules are then fed into the mitochondrial respiratory chain at Complex 3. As well as producing acetyl CoA the β-oxidation cycle directly reduces 1 molecule of FAD and NAD+ for each acetyl CoA produced. The four enzyme cycle of β-oxidation includes a acyl-CoA dehydrogenase (AD), a enoyl-CoA hydratase, a NAD^+-dependent dehydrogenase and a thiolase (Figure 7.9). There are several versions of each of these enzymes which are designed to deal with fatty acids of long, medium or short chain length. Long chain AD (LCAD) is located on the inner mitochondrial membrane. The remaining three long chain specific β-oxidation enzymes form a tri-functional complex also located on the inner membrane. The medium and short chain β-oxidation enzymes are located in the mitochondrial matrix electrons produced by β-oxidation are transferred to the mitochondrial respiratory chain through a variety of electron transferring flavoproteins (Figure 7.2).

Clinical features

Unlike glycolysis, β-oxidation requires aerobic conditions. It is important for skeletal and cardiac muscle function and is also vital for hepatic ketone body production. Thus defects of β-oxidation can cause hepatic, cardiac or skeletal muscle disease. The hepatic and cardiac manifestations usually have a neonatal or infantile onset and in that setting dominate the clinical picture. Hepatic involvement, which may be episodic, manifests as an acute hepatic encephalopathy with a fasting hypoglycaemia, hypoketonaemia and raised plasma free fatty acids. Acute cardiomyopathy can be accompanied by hepatic encephalopathy or by skeletal muscle involvement. In neonates and infants skeletal muscle involvement is usually manifest as generalised hypotonia with weakness and failure to thrive. In adults skeletal muscle involvement can present with a progressive lipid storage myopathy, or an acute failure of muscle energy production with muscle pain and myoglobinuria. Presentation with exercise induced myoglobinuria is particularly associated with muscle carnitine parmitoyl transferase (CPT) deficiency. Carnitine and most acyl-CoA dehydrogenase deficiencies are associated with a progressive lipid storage myopathy. There may be intra-familial variation in the clinical presentation of the same β-oxidation defect

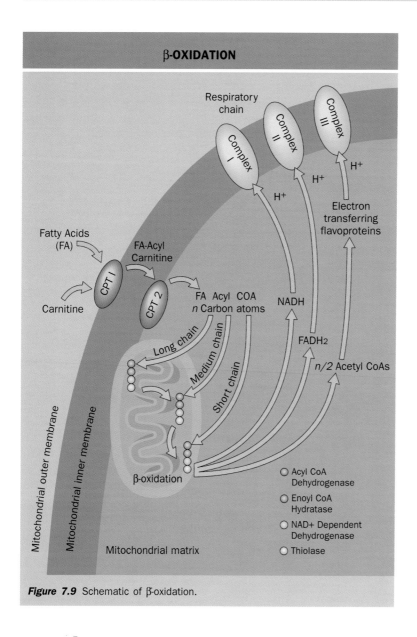

β-OXIDATION

Figure 7.9 Schematic of β-oxidation.

with different members having myopathic, cardiac or hepatic involvement (Table 7.9).

Carnitine deficiency

Carnitine deficiency is most often secondary to defects of β-oxidation or of the mitochondrial respiratory chain and can also be induced by sodium valproate and other drugs. Primary carnitine deficiency is rare and can be of the systemic, cardiac or muscle variety. The muscle involvement is one of a progressive muscle weakness with wasting and muscle biopsy showing accumulation of lipid particularly in type 1 fibres. There is usually an associated cardiomyopathy, encephalopathy or both.

The low blood and tissue carnitine levels seen in these conditions appear to be due to a defect in carnitine transport, certainly in the gut and kidney but possibly also in the cardiac and skeletal muscle. Inheritance is generally autosomal recessive with mutations in a sodium ion dependant carnitine transporter.

Carnitine palmitoyl transferase deficiency

Carnitine palmitoyl transferase deficiency occurs in three forms; muscle, hepatic and hepatomuscular CPT deficiency. Muscle CPT deficiency is due to a defect of CPT 2 and is one of the commonest defects of β-oxidation. It is more frequently seen in young adult males

Table 7.9 Defects of fatty acid metabolism

Enzyme/cofactor	Defect	Features
Fatty acid transport		
Carnitine	Primary carnitine deficiency	
Myopathic	Progressive lipid myopathy
Cardiac	Dilated cardiomyopathy +/- hepatic encephalopathy
Systemic	Hepatic encephalopathy and lipid myopathy
	Secondary carnitine deficiency	
Carnitine palmitoyl transferase 1 & 2	CPT deficiency	
	CPT 2 – Myopathic	Exercise induced myoglobinuria
	CPT 1 – Hepatic	Hepatic encephalopathy
	CPT 2 – Hepatomuscular	Severe infantile hypotonia and hepatic encephalopathy
Carnitine-acylcarnitine transferase	CT deficiency	Single case of hepatic encephalopathy, cardiomyopathy and myopathy
β oxidation		
Acyl-CoA dehydrogenase (AD)		
Long chain AD (LCAD) >12 C length	LCAD deficiency	Hepatic encephalopathy +/– lipid myopathy and myoglobinuria
Medium chain AD (MCAD) 4–14 C length	MCAD deficiency	Hepatic encephalopathy +/– lipid myopathy
Short chain AD (SCAD) 4–6 C length	SCAD deficiency	Lipid myopathy +/– hepatic encephalopathy
Enoyl-CoA hydratase		
Long chain and Short chain		
NAD+dependent dehydrogenase		Hepatic manifestations
Long chain and Short chain		
Thiolases		
Long chain specific and General thiolase		
Enzymes in italics form a tri-functional complex	Tri-functional enzyme deficiency	Hepatic encephalopathy +/– lipid myopathy and myoglobinuria
Electron transferring flavoproteins (ETF)		
Various		Hepatic encephalopathy +/– myopathy

perhaps because they tend to exercise harder. It results in symptoms of muscle pain and attacks of rhabdomyolysis with myoglobinuria. Attacks are typically triggered by prolonged exercise in fasting conditions but can also occur with intercurrent illness, fever and other biological stresses. Mild inter-ictal weakness can occur. It is an autosomal recessive disorder with missense mutations of the *CPT* gene located on chromosome 1p13.11. Hepatic CPT deficiency due to CPT 1 deficiency, and hepatomuscular CPT due to CPT 2 deficiency are much rarer and have an infantile onset with hepatic symptoms dominating.

LCAD deficiency

This can present with a similar clinical picture to medium chain acyl-CoA dehydrogenase (MCAD) deficiency (described below) but with earlier onset, more frequent attacks and higher morbidity. Muscle involvement is one of a lipid storage myopathy. There is a alternative presentation with more prominent muscle symptoms similar to CPT 2 deficiency namely muscle pain, weakness and myoglobinuria. Patients with very long chain acyl-CoA dehydrogenase deficiency also present like CPT 2 deficiency.

MCAD deficiency

This is the most common β-oxidation defect. The full range of symptoms are those associated with hepatic involvement precipitated by fasting, including nausea, vomiting, hypoglycaemia and hypoketonaemia leading to coma. Disease expression can be variable with some affected subjects being asymptomatic. There is a myopathic variant presenting with a mild lipid storage myopathy. 90% of cases with MCAD deficiency are associated with a homozygous recessive point mutation in the MCAD gene on chromosome 1p31.

SCAD deficiency

Short chain acyl-CoA dehydrogenase (SCAD) deficiency is rare but may have myopathic features alone with muscle wasting and weakness and massive lipid excess seen on muscle biopsy.

Investigations
General

Hepatic involvement results in hypoglycaemia, hypoketonaemia, hyperammonaemia and elevated transaminases. In addition there may be a dicarboxylic aciduria. Muscle involvement with acute rhabdomyolysis will result in a high CK and myoglobinuria but between attacks CK may be normal. Investigations may also reveal cardiomegaly with ECG abnormalities due to cardiomyopathy. Urinary organic acids may show a pattern of dicarboxylic acids which is specific for a given β-oxidation defect, but there may be no organic aciduria when the patient is well and normoglycaemic.

As many of the biochemical abnormalities of β oxidation may disappear between attacks a provocation test may be useful. The provocation is that of a prolonged fast, usually of at least 18 hours, sufficient to provoke the hypoglycaemia seen in β-oxidation defects or else produce ketonaemia if there is no β-oxidation defect. As this test carries the risk of provoking major biochemical upset including myoglobinuria it requires close and experienced monitoring. The safest screening test is tandem mass spectrometry on a blood sample taken after an overnight fast.

Muscle biopsy

In the lipid storage myopathies muscle biopsy stained with Sudan Black or Oil Red O may show an accumulation of lipid droplets especially in type 1 fibres. In cases where exercise induced pain with rhabdomyolysis is the main feature the muscle biopsy is usually normal except during or following attacks when fibre necrosis and lipid excess may be seen.

Specific biochemistry

In primary carnitine deficiency total and free serum carnitine is usually less than 10% of normal. Carnitine levels may however be low secondary to any β-oxidation defect with the exception of CPT 1 deficiency. In primary carnitine deficiency there is reduced carnitine uptake in cultured fibroblasts.

In carnitine parmitoyl transferase (CPT) deficiency the defect in muscle may be total or partial. The deficiency is also present in blood and skin samples.

Partial identification of the β-oxidation defect may be obtained by measuring 14C-labelled fatty acids in cultured fibroblasts and separating out the products so that the site of accumulation of fatty acid products can be determined. Measurement of individual β-oxidation enzymes is a technical challenge.

Molecular biology

This may become the easiest way to diagnose specific β-oxidation defects and is already of value in MCAD and CPT deficiency.

Management

General treatment

The mainstay of treatment is the prevention of prolonged fasting and patients should be on a low fat diet which should contain sufficient carbohydrate to maintain glucose levels while not provoking lipid storage. Extra carbohydrate may be required during intercurrent illness if necessary by tube or intravenous routes if oral intake is impossible or insufficient. In cases of LCAD deficiency with normal MCAD activity a diet containing medium chain fatty acids can circumvent the metabolic block.

Specific treatment

In primary carnitine deficiency, oral carnitine supplementation can be extremely helpful leading to restoration of normal cardiac function and improvement in the other clinical features. This treatment is less effective in secondary carnitine deficiencies.

Selected further reading

Angelini C, Vergani L, Martinuzzi A. Clinical and biochemical aspects of carnitine deficiency and insufficiency: transport defects and inborn errors of beta-oxidation. *Crit Rev Clin Lab Sci* 1992; 29: 217–242.

Di Donato S. Disorders of lipid metabolism in muscle. In: Engel AG, Franzini-Armstrong C (eds). *Myology* 2nd edn. New York: McGraw-Hill, 1994: 1587–1609.

Hammans SR, Sweeney MG, Holt IJ et al. Evidence for intramitochondrial complementation between deleted and normal mitochondrial DNA in some patients with mitochondrial myopathy. *J Neurol Sci* 1992; 107: 87–92.

Holt IJ, Harding AE, Morgan-Hughes JA. Deletions of muscle mitochondrial DNA in patients with mitochondrial myopathies. *Nature* 1998; 331: 717–719.

MITOMAP: A Human Mitochondrial Genome Database. Center for Molecular Medicine, Emory University, Atlanta, GA, USA, 2000. *http://www.gen.emory.edu/mitomap.html*

Morgan-Hughes J. Mitochondrial diseases. In: Engel AG, Franzini-Armstrong C (eds). *Myology* 2nd edn. New York: McGraw-Hill, 1994: 1610–1660.

Mullie MA, Harding AE, Petty RKH et al. The retinal manifestations of mitochondrial myopathy. *Arch Ophthalmol* 1985; 103: 1825–1830.

Nashef L, Lane RJM. Screening for mitochondrial cytopathies: the subanaerobic threshold exercise test (SATET). *J Neurol Neurosurg Psychiatry* 1989; 52: 1090–1094.

Rose MR. Mitochondrial myopathy; genetic mechanisms. *Arch Neurol* 1998; 55: 17–24.

Schapira AHV, Di Mauro S. *Mitochondrial Disorders in Neurology*. Oxford: Butterworth Heinemann, 1994.

Zierz S. Carnitine palmitoyltransferase deficiency. In: Engel AG, Franzini-Armstrong C (eds). *Myology* 2nd edn. New York: McGraw-Hill, 1994: 1577–1586.

chapter 8

Disorders of carbohydrate metabolism affecting muscle

The disorders to be discussed in this chapter are sometimes included in a chapter with headings such as "Glycogen Storage Diseases of Muscle", or "Muscle Glycogenoses". The former ignores the fact that in many of the conditions to be considered there is no glycogen excess in muscle. Both ignore the fact that many of these conditions are disorders of glycolysis rather than of glycogen metabolism. The broad remit of this chapter is inherited disorders of glycogen breakdown (glycogenolysis) and synthesis, and of glycolysis (Figure 8.1). Apart from muscle the other major site of glycogen metabolism is the liver, where it plays a vital role in gluconeogenesis, and some diseases have both hepatic and muscle manifestations. Others, because of the existence of muscle-specific isoenzymes, have only a myopathic component. Excluding acid maltase deficiency, the most commonly encountered purely muscle disorder is myophosphorylase deficiency (McArdle's disease), and the commonest affecting muscle and liver is debrancher enzyme deficiency. Acid maltase deficiency stands apart, clinically and biochemically, from the other conditions under discussion. It is a lysosomal rather than cytosolic enzyme (Figure 8.1), its normal role in metabolism is unclear, and the clinical features differ markedly depending upon the age of onset. It is not associated with exercise intolerance.

MAJOR ASPECTS OF GLYCOGEN AND GLUCOSE METABOLISM IN MUSCLE

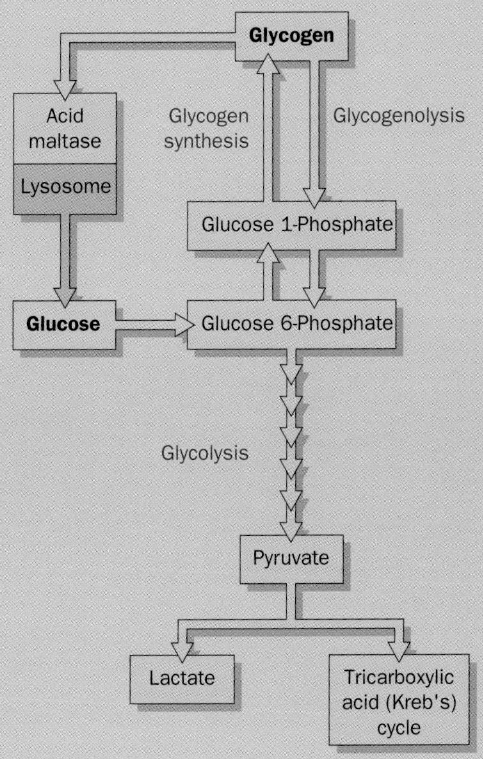

Figure 8.1 Major aspects of glycogen and glucose metabolism in muscle.

As a generalisation about the conditions to be discussed in this chapter, two major myopathic presentations are seen. Firstly, the patient may complain of exercise intolerance. This generally takes the form of exercise-induced weakness and cramps. More intense exercise may lead to muscle fibre breakdown with release of myoglobin into the circulation and the risk of renal failure caused by myoglobinuria. It is presumed, but not yet clearly proven, that these events are consequent upon a critical failure of energy metabolism. Secondly, there may be slowly progressive, exercise-unrelated, weakness. This is typically proximal in distribution, and mimics other causes of proximal myopathy such as the muscular dystrophies, but more rarely may be predominantly distal. Again, the precise mechanism is uncertain but may be due to glycogen accumulation causing disruption of muscle fibre structure and function. In some disorders both myopathic features are present, progressive weakness then usually developing after a long history of exercise intolerance.

Therapeutic approaches remain very limited. Rather than discuss them with respect to each of the disorders being considered, a final section is devoted to treatment principles.

Metabolic pathways

The role of glycogen and glucose metabolism in muscle energetics, and the relationship to fatty acid metabolism, was discussed in Chapter 2 (Exercise Tests). In brief summary, glycogen stored within muscle fibres is the major fuel during early, and particularly during intense, exercise. With long-duration sub-maximal exercise, increased blood flow leads to increased delivery of oxygen and fatty acids (mobilised from the body's lipid stores) to muscle, and fatty acids, through oxidative phosphorylation, become the main fuel for energy production. At rest, fatty acids are also the predominant source of the relatively limited energetic demands of muscle, and glucose entering muscle fibres is stored in glycogen for later use.

An outline of glycogen and glucose metabolism in muscle was shown in Figure 8.1. A more detailed description of glycogen synthesis and breakdown (glycogenolysis), and of glycolysis is given in Figures 8.2 and 8.3 respectively. Some of the major features of these pathways can be summarised as follows:

- Glycogen, not glucose, is the major source of fuel for glycolysis. During exercise some blood-borne glucose entering muscle undergoes glycolysis but at rest most is stored as glycogen for later use.
- Glycogen is a glucose polymer composed of tens of thousands of glucose molecules (Figure 8.4). The basic linear structure depends upon α-1,4 links between glucose units, whereas the branches are formed by α-1,6 links. Myophosphorylase (with inorganic phosphate) catalyzes the removal of a terminal glucose (linked by an α-1,4 bond) forming glucose 1-phosphate, which can enter glycolysis. Myophosphorylase can not cleave the α-1,6 links and so the action of myophosphorylase alone is to produce a pruned molecule known as limit dextrin. The α-1,6 links are the hydrolysed by debrancher enzyme following which myophosphorylase can continue to act on the newly exposed ends of the molecule. Thus, complete degradation of glycogen requires both myophosphorylase and debrancher enzyme activity. Myophosphorylase deficiency typically produces more severe exercise-induced

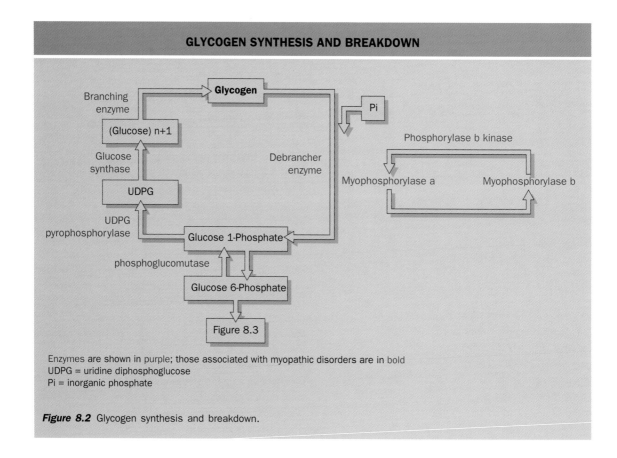

GLYCOGEN SYNTHESIS AND BREAKDOWN

Enzymes are shown in purple; those associated with myopathic disorders are in bold
UDPG = uridine diphosphoglucose
Pi = inorganic phosphate

Figure 8.2 Glycogen synthesis and breakdown.

GLYCOLYSIS

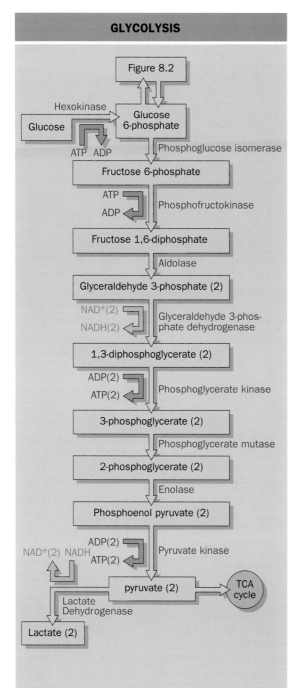

Figure 8.3 Glycolysis. Enzymes are shown in red; those associated with myopathic disorders are shown in bold type. ATP consuming and producing reactions are shown in blue. NADH consuming and producing reactions are shown in green. TCA = tricarboxylic acid cycle. See text for further discussion.

symptoms than debrancher enzyme deficiency because in the latter case normal myophosphorylase activity can release at least some of the glucose subunits from glycogen.

- Glycolysis alone is an inefficient producer of ATP, but under anaerobic conditions it is the only substantial source of ATP (a small amount is available from the creatine kinase reaction). The conversion of one molecule of glucose, derived from glycogen, to pyruvate generates a net three molecules of ATP. Glucose metabolism consumes an additional molecule of ATP so the net ATP production from glucose entering muscle directly is only two molecules. By contrast, under aerobic conditions the complete metabolism of a single molecule of glucose derived from glycogen generates 39 molecules of ATP; pyruvate enters the tricarboxylic acid cycle and reducing equivalents from here and from glycolysis are transferred to the mitochondrial respiratory chain.

- Under anaerobic conditions (e.g. early exercise) NADH generated by glyceraldehyde 3–phosphate dehydrogenase can not be re-oxidised to NAD^+ via the respiratory chain. Instead, NAD^+ is regenerated by the lactate dehydrogenase reaction. A characteristic feature of disorders carbohydrate metabolism in muscle is the impaired production of lactate during exercise and this forms the basis of the ischaemic forearm exercise test (see Chapter 2). The failure of acidification can be demonstrated by phosphorus magnetic resonance spectroscopy. Conversely, mitochondrial disorders are often associated with excessive lactate production which may be demonstrated, for example, by bicycle ergometry.

- Acid maltase is not involved in ATP generation. This lysosomal enzyme can cleave both α-1,4 and α-1,6 bonds.

Those enzymes known to be associated with myopathic disorders are shown in Figures 8.2 and 8.3. The disorders of terminal glycolysis (deficiencies of phosphoglycerate kinase, phosphoglycerate mutase, and lactate dehydrogenase) have been described only recently and are very much rarer than myophosphorylase and debrancher enzyme deficiency. It is probable that there are other muscle glycogenoses yet to be identified.

Disorders of glycogenolysis

The most important of these disorders (Figure 8.2) are acid maltase deficiency, myophosphorylase deficiency

GLYCOGEN

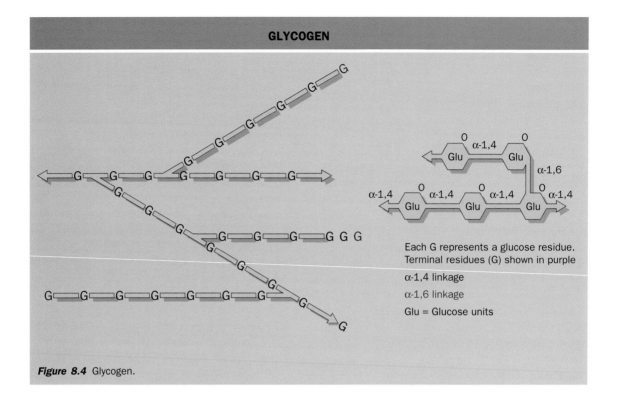

Each G represents a glucose residue.
Terminal residues (G) shown in purple

α-1,4 linkage
α-1,6 linkage
Glu = Glucose units

Figure 8.4 Glycogen.

and debrancher enzyme deficiency. Some of the unique aspects of acid maltase deficiency have already been noted. Myophosphorylase deficiency presents as a myopathic disorder, although its recognition is often very delayed. Even within a specialist muscle clinic it is uncommon. One of our clinics, with a catchment population of over 2 million people, sees about one new case every two years. The figure for adult-onset acid maltase deficiency is similar. Debrancher enzyme deficiency is typically first recognised in childhood because of hepatic features. Such patients may later develop a myopathy. Less frequently, presentation is in late-childhood or adult life with a proximal myopathy, but we see this even less often than new cases of myophosphorylase deficiency. The other two conditions, phosphorylase b kinase deficiency and phosphoglucomutase deficiency, are rarer still.

Acid maltase deficiency

Synonyms: Glycogen storage disease type II, Pompe's disease, acid α-glucosidase deficiency.

As already noted, acid maltase is not part of the glycolytic pathway and so exercise-intolerance, which is a typical feature of the conditions discussed later, is not apparent.

Clinical features

Although there is some overlap, most cases fall readily into one of three categories: infantile, childhood and adult forms. Skeletal muscle involvement is present in all three types and is the predominant, and indeed typically the only, feature in adult-onset cases.

Infantile form

This is the form of the condition that Pompe described and it is characterised by enormous glycogen excess in many organs. Onset is within the first few months of life. The major clinical features are hypotonia and weakness, cardiomyopathy, macroglossia, hepatomegaly and respiratory failure. Death occurs within two years from cardiorespiratory failure. Hypoglycaemia, seen in many of the hepatic glycogenoses, is not a feature because of the metabolic position of acid maltase.

Childhood form

This form presents as a myopathy and is an important differential diagnosis to muscular dystrophy. Serum creatine kinase is elevated. It may cause delayed motor milestones or present later, but always before the age of 15 years. As in the adult form there may be selective involvement of respiratory muscles. Visceromegaly is infrequent. Death, in the second or third decade of life, is usually due to cardiorespiratory failure.

Adult form

Largely because clinical expression is almost invariably confined to skeletal muscle, this is the form that is of greatest interest to myologists. Onset is after the age of 20 years, sometimes not until late-middle age, and broadly speaking it presents in one of two ways. The typical presentation is with a slowly progressive proximal myopathy that is clinically indistinguishable from many other causes of limb-girdle syndrome (e.g. other metabolic myopathies, dystrophies, inflammatory myopathies). The more dramatic presentation, which may be seen in up to one-third of cases, is with respiratory failure. Although the symptoms may not have been acted upon, such patients typically have a short history of nocturnal respiratory insufficiency with disturbed sleep pattern, headaches on waking and excessive daytime sleepiness. Most also have some symptoms suggestive of long-standing muscle weakness. In those presenting with proximal weakness, a close eye must be kept on their respiratory function over the following years. Respiratory muscle weakness is often very satisfactorily dealt with using night-time positive pressure ventilation applied via a face mask.

One of our patients exemplifies many of the features of adult-onset acid maltase deficiency. In his mid-twenties he was referred by his general practitioner to an orthopaedic surgeon because of an abnormal gait and the suspicion of hip disease. Further assessment showed pelvic girdle weakness and investigations were initiated. He woke one morning and was noted to be drowsy and confused. The ambulance crew found him to be cyanosed and put on an oxygen mask which precipitated respiratory failure. Subsequently a history of recent morning headaches and daytime sleepiness was elicited. He was mechanically ventilated for a short time but was then successfully weaned and eventually required only nocturnal ventilatory support with a positive pressure ventilator and face mask. The diagnosis of acid maltase deficiency was established. He was able to return to full-time work for many years.

The weak muscles are atrophic in proportion to the weakness. Occasionally there is remarkably selective involvement of certain muscles, mimicking some of the muscular dystrophies. Tendon reflexes are lost as a late feature. Respiratory failure is due to diaphragmatic weakness and this may be evident at the bedside in the form of paradoxical movement of the upper abdomen on inspiration (see Chapter 1). Clinical assessment alone is insufficient. The forced vital capacity (FVC) should routinely be measured with the patient lying and standing. With weakness of the diaphragm the FVC increases on standing because of the descent of the abdominal contents. Radiological screening may show impaired movement of the diaphragm. A more sensitive, but not readily repeatable, test is to measure the transdiaphragmatic pressure using oesophageal balloons.

Non-myopathic features are very uncommon in adult-onset cases, although it is reasonable to periodically assess the cardiac status (ECG and echocardiography). Hepatomegaly and macroglossia are very rare. Although they may be coincidental, there have been reports of intracranial vascular malformations apparently directly related to the disorder (glycogen excess has been shown in smooth muscle). Indeed, the patient described above was found to have a small frontal lobe arteriovenous malformation.

Diagnosis

This is relatively straightforward. The serum creatine kinase is always elevated in the infantile and childhood forms and usually elevated in adult-onset cases. Electromyography shows "myopathic" features (short-duration polyphasic motor unit potentials) but in addition frequently present, and a hint towards the diagnosis, are features of muscle fibre irritability with repetitive discharges including myotonic discharges, fibrillation potentials, and positive sharp waves.

Glycogen accumulates in lymphocytes and this may be shown on an air-dried blood film treated with celloidin and stained with periodic acid Schiff (PAS) reagent (Figure 8.5). This is a sensitive and specific test for all forms of acid maltase deficiency.

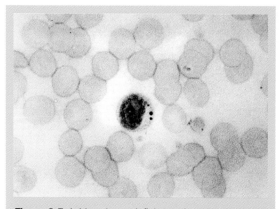

Figure 8.5 Acid maltase deficiency. Lymphocyte glycogen storage (periodic acid-Schiff stain). The darkly staining glycogen granules are readily apparent.

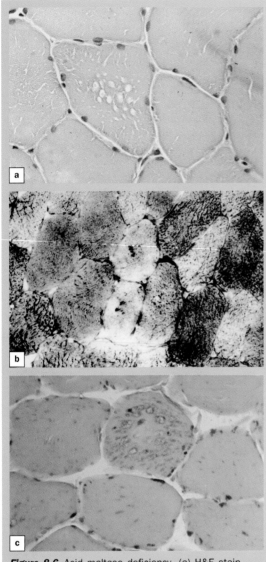

Figure 8.6 Acid maltase deficiency. (a) H&E stain. Note the vacuoles which, on PAS staining (b), are shown to contain glycogen and stain for acid phosphatase (c).

Muscle biopsy shows a vacuolar myopathy (Figure 8.6). The changes are more severe in the earlier onset form and it is very important to note that in adult-onset cases the biopsy may be normal histologically. The vacuoles contain glycogen, which stains with PAS. The vacuoles also stain for acid phosphatase indicating their lysosomal origin. Increased acid phosphatase activity in the absence of vacuoles may also be a pointer to the diagnosis.

Although the lymphocyte changes are specific, the diagnosis is often confirmed by enzyme assay. This can be done on liver, leucocytes and cultured fibroblasts, but as muscle is often available this is the commonest substrate for the assay. There is a poor correlation between clinical severity and residual enzyme activity and with the presence or absence of immunoreactive material.

Genetics and molecular biology

It is inherited as an autosomal recessive disorder. Mutations have been identified in the acid maltase gene, located at 17q23–25. Studies in cultured fibroblasts have shown a variety of biochemical abnormalities including reduced enzyme precursor synthesis, defective phosphorylation of the enzyme and abnormal processing. To date, no simple correlation between the genotype or biochemical defect, and the phenotype has emerged. Similarly, there is no correlation between the type of clinical presentation and the amount of residual enzyme activity measured in muscle.

Myophosphorylase deficiency

Synonyms: Glycogen storage disease type V, McArdle's disease.

The clinical features, and the characteristic failure to produce lactate on ischaemic exercise, were delineated by McArdle in 1951. He deduced that there was an enzyme defect in the pathway of glycogen breakdown, but it was not until 1959 that the absence of muscle phosphorylase (myophosphorylase) was identified. As myophosphorylase is a tissue-specific enzyme, confined to skeletal and cardiac muscle, the systemic manifestations seen with many of the other glycogenoses are absent.

Clinical features

The characteristic feature of this condition is exercise intolerance. Although the age of onset is typically before the age of 20 years, and often in the first decade of life, the diagnosis is frequently not made until much later. For example, two of our recent cases did not seek medical attention until their 50s despite a history of symptoms clearly dating back to their school-days. An informal survey found the average age of diagnosis to be 28 years of age. There is an excess of male cases, the cause of which is not established, but for which suggestions have included hormonal factors and differing levels of physical activity.

Symptoms develop early in the course of exercise, and sooner the more intense the activity. Muscle pain is accompanied by weakness and stiffness. The latter may be seen as inability to fully extend the fingers after vigorous finger flexion. Severe stiffness results in a contracture that superficially resembles a true muscle cramp. However, the contracture is electrically silent whereas of course cramps are caused by excessive motor nerve activity.

Muscle damage occurs during exercise. If this is extensive then myoglobinuria results, with the risk of renal failure (See Chapter 1 – Myoglobinuria). Some two-thirds of patients will at some time during their life experience an episode of myoglobinuria, but it is rare in childhood and adolescence. Of these, up to one-quarter will develop renal failure. Because pain precedes muscle damage sufficient to cause myoglobinuria, most patients learn to limit their exercise to safe limits. This is often a subconscious process in that they will learn this even before presenting for medical assessment.

The degree of exercise intolerance varies enormously. A few patients have such severe exercise-intolerance that they spend much of their time wheelchair-bound, but this is unusual. Most lead fairly normal lives, as long as they avoid strenuous exercise and rest or reduce the level of activity when myalgia develops. A recent patient presented with myoglobinuria (and a creatine kinase level of over 100,000 IU/l) after playing squash for 80 minutes. He had played squash nearly every week of his adult life and in retrospect had noticed that it took him longer to warm up than his partner, but thereafter he played an effective game! Previously he had never played for more than 40 minutes.

The patient described above demonstrates vividly the "second-wind" phenomenon. As noted in Chapter 2 (Metabolic changes during exercise) and above, energy demands in early exercise are met by anaerobic glycogenolysis and glycolysis. In myophosphorylase deficiency glycogenolysis is defective, hence the symptoms at the start of physical activity. As exercise continues aerobic fatty acid oxidation becomes the main source of energy and this process is normal in patients with defects of glycogenolysis and glycolysis. Patients often learn, again apparently subconsciously, that if they lower their exercise rate at the onset of discomfort they can then carry on for longer, having developed the "second-wind". If they have not identified this process for themselves then it is an important part of their management to educate them about it.

A proportion of patients, perhaps one-third, develop progressive proximal weakness which may be accompanied by mild wasting. Rarely, such patients do not in addition have typical exercise-induced symptoms and they may thus mimic many other causes of proximal myopathy. We have seen a number of patients, with typical exercise-related symptoms, with persistent asymptomatic weakness of neck flexion in the absence of weakness elsewhere.

Myophosphorylase is present in cardiac muscle, but is only one of several isoenzymes. Cardiac involvement is generally not considered to be a feature of myophosphorylase deficiency. We have seen exercise-induced chest pain in a few patients without evidence, on detailed investigation, of ischaemic heart disease. The pain probably arises from the chest wall muscles.

Epilepsy has been commented upon in some reports but there is no certain link with myophosphorylase deficiency, although the enzyme is probably expressed in brain.

Some very atypical presentations have been reported, but all are rare. They include onset of typical exercise-related symptoms in late-middle age, progressive myopathy in adult life without exercise-related symptoms, an acute fatal infantile form and a milder congenital form, and childhood-onset progressive myopathy without exercise-related features.

Diagnosis

The serum creatine kinase is elevated in the vast majority of cases. Electromyography is often normal or shows only non-specific myopathic changes. Contractures are electrically silent, distinguishing them from cramp, but there is no value in seeking this finding and indeed it is hazardous to the patient.

A conventional approach to diagnosis is through the ischaemic forearm exercise test (see Chapter 2). The failure to generate lactate is common to many disorders of glycogenolysis and glycolysis, so the test is not specific to myophosphorylase deficiency. Sometimes, lactate generation is impaired rather than totally absent, resulting in a false-negative test. A very common finding is absent lactate generation due to lack of effort in patients with non-organic causes of myalgia. To detect this, ammonia is measured simultaneously with lactate (see Chapter 2, figure 2.7). For all of these reasons the value of the test is somewhat limited and it should only be performed in a specialist department. Another hazard, albeit rare, is the development of severe contracture of the forearm muscles, myoglobinuria and renal failure.

More valuable than the ischaemic forearm exercise test, but of limited availability, is phosphorus magnetic resonance spectroscopy (see Chapter 2). Advantages include the fact that the test is performed aerobically, measurement of phosphocreatine acts as an internal control (like ammonia) to make certain that the subject

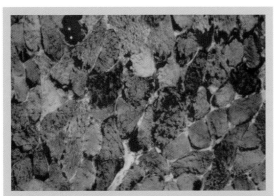

Figure 8.7 Myophosphorylase deficiency. Periodic acid-Schiff stain shows accumulation of glycogen, which may form "lakes".

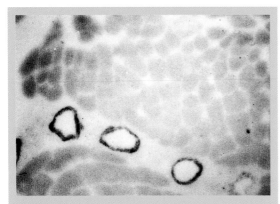

Figure 8.8 Myophosphorylase deficiency. The skeletal muscle fibres do not stain for phosphorylase, but the smooth muscle of blood vessels does, providing a useful internal control to show that the staining technique is working.

exercises adequately, and disorders of distal glycolysis results in the detection of phosphorylated intermediates of glycolysis.

In most cases the diagnosis is suspected clinically and confirmed on the basis of muscle biopsy findings. Subsarcolemmal glycogen accumulation is readily seen in most cases (Figure 8.7), although occasionally the changes are subtle. Phosphorylase staining is absent from muscle fibres (Figure 8.8), although regenerating fibres show staining and the smooth muscle of intramuscular blood vessels also stains (serving as an internal control that the stain is working). If further proof of the diagnosis is considered necessary then the enzyme activity can be assayed – residual activity is seen in up to one-quarter of cases.

Genetics and molecular biology

Myophosphorylase deficiency is inherited as an autosomal recessive disorder. Earlier reports suggesting dominant inheritance in some families are almost certainly explained upon the basis of compound heterozygotes. The myophosphorylase gene is located on chromosome 11q13. Several mutations have been described, the commonest being at codon 49 of exon 1 (R49X).

No clear correlation has yet emerged between the clinical picture and residual enzyme activity, amount of cross-immunoreactive material and mRNA levels.

Phosphorylase b kinase deficiency

Synonyms: Glycogen storage disease type VIa.

Myophosphorylase has active (myophosphorylase a) and inactive (myophosphorylase b) forms (Figure 8.2). Myophosphorylase b is phosphorylated to the active a-form by phosphorylase b kinase (which itself has an active phosphorylated and a less active non-phosphorylated form). Phosphorylase b kinase is present in all tissues and plays a key role in glycogen metabolism. The commonest presentation is as a relatively benign, X-linked, disorder with hepatomegaly and fasting hypoglycaemia, without muscle involvement. The second commonest form is inherited as an autosomal recessive condition. Hepatic involvement is similar to the X-linked form but in addition there is hypotonia in infancy and mild non-progressive weakness later. Those rarer presentations with more significant cardioskeletal muscle involvement are discussed below.

Clinical features

Several patients have been described with exercise-induced muscle pain and stiffness, and myoglobinuria, presenting in childhood and early adult life. Progressive proximal weakness has been described, as has predominantly distal progressive weakness in the absence of exercise-induced symptoms. These patients do not have cardiac involvement. Another form of the disease consists of isolated cardiomegaly and death in early infancy.

Diagnosis

In the myopathic forms the serum creatine kinase is usually elevated. Electromyography may be normal or show features of primary muscle disease. The ischaemic exercise test may be normal or show impaired or absent lactate generation.

Muscle biopsy shows a vacuolar myopathy due to glycogen accumulation. Diagnosis is confirmed by enzyme assay on a muscle biopsy sample.

Genetics and molecular biology

Phosphorylase b kinase is a tetrameric structure composed of four sub-units, α, β, γ, and δ, coded on chromosomes X, 16, 17 and 7 respectively. The genetic and molecular basis of the various clinical presentations remains unclear, but a candidate gene for the commonest X-linked form has been identified.

Debrancher enzyme deficiency

Synonyms: Glycogen storage disease type III, Cori-Forbes disease, amylo-1,6-glucosidase deficiency.

Debrancher enzyme (Figure 8.2) is ubiquitously expressed without tissue-specific isoenzymes. Despite this, there are two distinct clinical presentations and several different patterns of molecular derangement. As noted, the enzyme is required for the complete breakdown of glycogen. In its absence, myophosphorylase can cleave terminal glucose residues, leaving a limit dextrin. Since some glucose can be released from glycogen, exercise-induced symptoms are less evident than in myophosphorylase deficiency.

Clinical features

Two main phenotypes are recognised. The commoner is with predominantly hepatic features presenting in childhood, the rarer is an adult presentation with myopathy.

Childhood presentation

Onset is typically in the first year of life with hypoglycaemia, seizures, failure to thrive and hepatomegaly. Infantile hypotonia and delayed motor milestones may or may not be noted. The hepatic features typically disappear around puberty. Some of these children have skeletal muscle enzyme deficiency and in them the myopathy progresses despite resolution of the liver problems. Others appear to have muscle enzyme activity and they do not have further problems.

Adult presentation

Although the presentation may not be until adulthood, many such patients have had asymptomatic hepatic involvement in childhood (a protuberant abdomen) and may also give a history of delayed motor milestones, poor athletic ability and difficulty in keeping up with their peers. A few patients have persistent hepatomegaly. There is slowly progressive weakness, usually proximal but sometimes distal, sometimes accompanied by muscle hypertrophy. Exercise intolerance is rarely severe and myoglobinuria is uncommon.

Cardiac involvement is very common, at least on investigation. However, sometimes dramatic ECG and echocardiographic changes may not be accompanied by cardiac symptoms. Regular assessment is required.

Diagnosis

In all forms of the disease, glucagon administration in the fasting state fails to produce a hyperglycaemic response. In the myopathic forms the serum creatine kinase is elevated. Electromyography shows features of primary muscle disease and, in addition, "irritable" features such as fibrillation potentials and complex repetitive discharges. Lactate generation during the ischaemic forearm exercise test is reduced or absent. The phosphorus magnetic resonance spectroscopy findings are indistinguishable from those of myophosphorylase deficiency.

Muscle biopsy shows a vacuolar myopathy with the glycogen-containing vacuoles typically subsarcolemmal in location.

The diagnosis is confirmed by enzyme assay. This can be on a muscle sample if it is available, or on red blood cells.

Genetics and molecular biology

The enzyme is a monomer and the gene is located on chromosome 1p21. It has two enzymatic activities; a transferase function shifts the glucose residues that remain after the action of myophosphorylase on to the outer end of another branch, and then a glucosidase function cleaves the α-1,6 linkage (Figure 8.4). Four patterns of residual activity in liver and muscle can be recognised, of which type IIIa is the commonest:

IIIa - Deficiency of both enzyme activities in liver and muscle.

IIIb - Deficiency of both enzyme activities in liver alone.

IIIc - Deficiency of both enzyme activities in muscle alone.

IIId - Deficiency of transferase activity, but normal glucosidase activity, in both liver and muscle.

Phosphoglucomutase deficiency

This is the only enzyme common to glycogen synthesis and degradation (Figure 8.2). Only a couple of cases have been described and they showed rather different clinical pictures. One had a mild myopathy. The other a Reye-like picture.

Disorders of glycolysis

Of the four known disorders (Figure 8.3) phosphofructokinase deficiency is by far the commonest, but even this has been reported in less than fifty patients, although there are certainly other unreported individuals. Haemolysis is an accompanying feature in some of these disorders, reflecting the importance of glycolysis in red cell metabolism. With the more distal defects of glycolysis muscle biopsy frequently does not show glycogen excess, either histologically or on assay.

Phosphofructokinase deficiency

Synonyms: Glycogen storage disease type VII, Tarui's disease.

Like myophosphorylase deficiency there is an excess of male cases, unexpected given the autosomal recessive pattern of inheritance. Most patients have come from Japanese or Ashkenazi Jewish backgrounds, but cases from Europe have been described. Phosphofructokinase plays a critical role in glycolysis (Figure 8.3) and unlike in the glycogenoses even circulating glucose cannot be utilised.

Some of the clinical variability is explained by the isoenzyme pattern. The enzyme is a tetramer formed from one or more sub-units. Muscle contains only M type, liver only L type, and erythrocytes various combinations of M and L.

Clinical features

Four broad groups can be identified. One, not to be discussed further, presents with haemolysis in the absence of skeletal muscle involvement.

The most typical presentation is with exercise-induced symptoms (weakness, cramps, contractures, myoglobinuria) similar to those seen in myophosphorylase deficiency. The age of onset is possibly earlier than in myophosphorylase deficiency, but even so diagnosis is typically delayed until adult life. The "second-wind phenomenon" has been reported only infrequently – perhaps because these patients, unlike those with a glycogenosis, are unable to utilise circulating glucose that enters muscle. Permanent muscle weakness in these patients is uncommon. In these patients there is almost invariably laboratory evidence of haemolysis but clinical sequelae are limited. About one-quarter have jaundice, rarely associated with gall stone formation. Asymptomatic hyperuricaemia is common but clinical gout infrequent. Hepatic uric acid production is increased due to enhanced activity of the myoadenylate deaminase pathway (Figure 2.7).

In a third group, reported in only half a dozen cases, onset is congenital or early infantile with weakness, respiratory insufficiency, mental retardation, epilepsy, cortical blindness and corneal damage.

The fourth, and apparently rarest group comprises late-adult onset of progressive weakness with a childhood history of easy fatigue but no cramps or myoglobinuria.

Diagnosis

The serum creatine kinase is almost invariably elevated and electromyography shows changes consistent with primary muscle disease as well as positive sharp waves, fibrillation potentials and pseudomyotonic discharges.

In most patient the ischaemic forearm exercise test shows impaired lactate generation. Magnetic resonance spectroscopy is more informative, showing failure of the pH to fall during exercise and accumulation of phosphorylated intermediates of glycolysis, the latter differentiating the condition from the glycogenolytic disorders.

Muscle biopsy shows glycogen accumulation and non-specific muscle fibre damage. Phosphofructokinase deficiency can be demonstrated histochemically but most cases have been confirmed by enzyme assay on a muscle biopsy sample. Significant residual enzyme activity may be seen in muscle. Red cell enzyme activity is typically 50% of normal.

Genetics and molecular biology

The tetrameric phosphofructokinase enzyme is composed of one, two or three different types of subunit. The M (muscle), L (liver) and P (platelet) subunits are encoded by genes on chromosomes 1, 21 and 10, respectively. Muscle contains the homotetramer M_4, liver the homotetramer L_4, and erythrocytes an admix of M_4, M_3L_1, M_2L_2, M_1L_3, and L_4. Myopathy results from mutations in the muscle phosphofructokinase gene. There is considerable genetic heterogeneity and no clear correlation between genotype and phenotype. Many mutations have been described and include mis-sense mutations and splicing defects. Two common mutations, the more frequent a splicing defect affecting exon 5, account for some two-thirds of Ashkenazi Jewish cases.

Phosphoglycerate kinase deficiency

Synonyms: Glycogen storage disease type IX.

A singular feature of this condition, compared with the other disorders discussed in this chapter, is that it is inherited as an X-liked disorder. There are no tissue-specific isoforms but some of the clinical variability can be explained upon the basis of genetic polymorphism. The commonest presentation is with haemolytic anaemia, without muscle involvement, often accompanied by central nervous system (epilepsy and mental retardation). Less than a dozen cases with skeletal muscle involvement have been reported.

Clinical features

The principal myopathic feature is exercise intolerance (cramps and myoglobinuria). In the limited reports permanent weakness appears uncommon. Additional features have included, chronic haemolysis, mental retardation, and retinitis pigmentosa.

Diagnosis

The serum creatine kinase and electromyography may be normal. Lactate generation during ischaemic exercise is impaired and phosphorus magnetic resonance spectroscopy, as in phosphofructokinase deficiency shows accumulation of sugar phosphates.

Muscle biopsy has shown minor, non-specific, myopathic features and glycogen content is normal.

The diagnosis is confirmed by enzyme assay on a muscle sample. Other tissues, such as red cells and fibroblasts, may be used but there is considerable variability in residual enzyme activity between different tissues.

Genetics and molecular biology

Different point mutations within the phosphoglycerate kinase (PGK) gene give rise to protein variants that can be identified on the basis of their electrophoretic mobility. Some variants are benign and asymptomatic (e.g. PGK München). Variants associated with myopathy include PGK Creteil, PGK New Jersey, PGK Hamamatsu, PGK Shizuoka, PGK Alberta, and PGK North Carolina.

Phosphoglycerate mutase deficiency

Synonyms: Glycogen storage disease type X.

This enzyme is a dimer formed from M (muscle) and B (brain) subunits. Myopathy has been reported in about ten patients, nearly all African Americans, and is associated with mutations of the M-sub-unit gene.

Clinical features

All reported patients have had exercise intolerance and renal failure secondary to myoglobinuria has been described. Permanent weakness doesn't appear to occur. One patient may have had cardiac involvement.

Diagnosis

Although the serum creatine kinase is typically elevated, electromyography and light microscopy have usually been normal. Lactate production during ischaemic exercise is impaired and phosphorus magnetic resonance spectroscopy shows changes of the type seen in phosphofructokinase and phosphoglycerate kinase deficiency.

The diagnosis is confirmed by enzyme assay on a muscle sample. Residual activity of up to 10% may be seen, reflecting MB and BB activity.

Genetics and molecular biology

Like all the disorders discussed in this chapter, except phosphoglycerate kinase deficiency, this glycogenosis is inherited as an autosomal recessive. The M sub-unit gene is on chromosome 7 and three different mutations have been identified. Disease may be associated with homozygous mutations or compound heterozygosity.

Lactate dehydrogenase deficiency

Synonyms: Glycogen storage disease type XI.

This is the rarest of the glycolytic disorders under discussion, with only a handful of patients having been described. It is inherited as an autosomal recessive. The enzyme is a tetramer composed of one or two types of sub-unit: M (muscle) also sometimes called A, and H (heart) sometimes called B.

Clinical features

Although an asymptomatic woman with lactate dehydrogenase (LDH) deficiency has been described, other patients have had typical exercise intolerance with myoglobinuria. Permanent or progressive weakness has not been described.

Diagnosis

Two interesting biochemical features may suggest the diagnosis. During the ischaemic forearm exercise test lactate generation is impaired but, in distinction to all of the conditions discussed earlier, a specific additional feature is the increase in the pyruvate:lactate ratio, readily understandable from the function of the enzyme (Figure 8.3). Secondly, following exercise the serum creatine kinase level rises but LDH does not, and indeed this observation was a pointer to the diagnosis in the first patient identified with LDH deficiency.

Muscle biopsy appearances have not been described. Residual enzyme activity in muscle is very low, confirming the diagnosis, but is near normal in red and white blood cells. Electrophoretic analysis shows absence of the M sub-unit band.

Genetics and molecular biology

The gene for the M sub-unit is on chromosome 11. Deletions involving 2 and 20 bases have been identified and a point mutation.

Disorders of glycogen synthesis

The only recognised disorder of glycogen synthesis (remember that the synthesis and breakdown pathways are different: Figure 8.2) is branching enzyme deficiency. It is a rare condition in which hepatic features predominate, but skeletal and cardiac muscle can be affected.

Branching enzyme deficiency

Synonyms: Glycogen storage disease type IV, polyglucosan body disease, Andersen's disease, amylopectinosis.

Branching enzyme inserts the α-1,6 branch points into the growing glycogen molecule (Figure 8.4). Its deficiency results in the accumulation of a glucose polymer (resembling amylopectin) referred to as polyglucosan, although this term is also used to describe a number of other structures including corpora amylacea and Lafora bodies.

Clinical features

The commonest presentation is in early infancy. The child appears normal at birth but within months develops gastrointestinal symptoms, hepatosplenomegaly, portal hypertension, ascites and cirrhosis. At least one-half of patients have hypotonia, muscular atrophy and depressed tendon reflexes. Untreated (treatment is by liver transplantation) death occurs, from liver failure, by the age of four years. At least one patient initially successfully treated by liver transplantation later died from cardiomyopathy.

Predominantly myopathic presentations are exceedingly rare. A few patients have been described presenting with progressive cardiomyopathy in adolescence and all had some degree of skeletal myopathy. Progressive skeletal myopathy as the primary problem has been reported only once.

Diagnosis

Massive accumulation of polyglucosan bodies is seen in many tissues including skeletal, smooth and cardiac muscle, sweat glands, axons and perineurial cells, astrocytes, and fibroblasts. Diagnosis is confirmed by enzyme assay in muscle. Patients have been described with cardioskeletal myopathy and polyglucosan body deposition, but with normal branching enzyme activity.

Genetics and molecular biology

Inheritance is autosomal recessive. The branching enzyme gene is on chromosome 3 and has recently been cloned. Prenatal diagnosis by enzyme assay on fibroblasts cultured from amniotic fluid cells is possible.

Therapeutic aspects

Unfortunately, therapeutic advances, especially with respect to treatment of myopathic features, have advanced less spectacularly than our knowledge of molecular mechanisms. Although specific treatments are lacking, that is not to say that no therapeutic options are available and indeed a great deal can be done to help these patients. In several of the glycogenoses hepatic involvement is common and of major clinical significance. A number of therapeutic strategies may be effective, depending upon the site of the enzyme defect. Thus, in debrancher enzyme deficiency in childhood high-protein nocturnal enteral therapy improves exercise tolerance, muscle strength and growth rate.

Specific therapies for the skeletal and cardiac muscle involvement in individual disorders are almost certainly still some way off. Attempts, so far unsuccessful, to treat acid maltase deficiency in patients have included enzyme replacement by intravenous injection and bone marrow transplantation. More encouragingly, intravenous injection of recombinant human acid α-glucosidase into acid maltase-deficient quail not only improved biochemical parameters, but also substantially improved muscle function so that birds that couldn't lift their wings were able to fly. No specific (i.e. enzyme replacement) therapies have yet emerged for the major glycogenolytic and glycolytic disorders. Branching enzyme deficiency in early infancy responds to liver transplantation, a remarkable feature being that extra-hepatic amylopectin deposition, including that in skeletal and cardiac muscle, also reduces.

Respiratory involvement is a late feature in most of the disorders considered in this chapter, only developing when there is extensive limb weakness. The striking exception is acid maltase deficiency in which up to one-third of patients present in respiratory failure, and for some considerable time have no significant limb weakness. Such patients are particularly satisfying to treat because they can return to a near-enough normal existence, including full-time work. Although a number of techniques have been used, such as rocking-beds and cuirass ventilators, by far the most effective and patient-acceptable is positive pressure nocturnal ventilation using a face mask.

Cardiomyopathy may be an early or a late feature. It appears to be very common in the adolescent/early-adult form of debrancher enzyme deficiency but sometimes the dramatic findings on ECG and echocardiography are not paralleled by major clinical problems. Close follow-up is required and the prognosis and best approaches to management remain to be determined.

Much has been written concerning exercise and diet. In those conditions associated with exercise-induced rhabdomyolysis, such as myophosphorylase deficiency, it is common sense to advise patients to try to avoid exercise strenuous enough to precipitate such a problem, although many of them will already have learnt this for themselves. It also seems reasonable also to advise regular low-intensity exercise to improve the oxidative capacity of muscle and thus to enhance the "second-wind" phenomenon. Whereas dietary manipulation is undoubtedly helpful for the hepatic aspects of some disorders, the benefits with respect to skeletal muscle are less certain and remain somewhat controversial.

In myophosphorylase deficiency numerous attempts have been made to improve symptoms either by encouraging glucose metabolism, through the administration of glucose, fructose or glucagon, or by providing an alternative fuel in the form of a high-fat diet or by lipid infusion. Although some improvement in exercise tolerance, particularly in the short term, has been shown, long-term benefit and patient acceptability is poor and none can be recommended for routine practice.

The place for a high-protein diet (>25% of calories provided as protein) has its proponents but remains somewhat controversial, and in our experience is of limited benefit. In some of those studies claiming substantial benefit, it may well have been the coexistent exercise programme that provided the major benefit. That is not to undermine the very real benefits to patients of offering a comprehensive management package in which they are an active participant. The rationale behind such a dietary approach is at least two-fold. Firstly, some amino acids, particularly branched-chain ones, may be used directly by muscle for energy generation. Secondly, in the disease situation, amino acids may be used as an alternative energy source by muscle, thus reducing their availability for protein synthesis, which may then contribute towards the myopathy. Many patients find such a high-protein diet unpalatable and unless the total calorie content is carefully monitored weight gain can be a problem. It is certainly reasonable to suggest such dietary manipulations, and for the trial to last a reasonable period of time (say, 6 months) but in our experience the benefits are limited. Advice concerning a suitable exercise regime is probably as important.

Although not a treatment for a specific disorder, it is appropriate to comment on the treatment of myoglobinuria, which is a serious complication of several of the disorders mentioned here, as well as in other metabolic myopathies such as carnitine palmitoyltransferase deficiency. It is presumed that renal damage occurs as a result of deposition of myoglobin. Treatment is by forced alkaline diuresis, on the principle that dehydration and acidosis enhance myoglobin precipitation. Dialysis is required if renal failure develops.

Selected further reading

General textbooks and reviews

DiMauro S, Bruno C. Glycogen storage diseases of muscle. *Curr Opin Neurol* 1998; 11: 477–484.

Engel AG, Franzini-Armstrong C (eds). *Myology* 2nd edn. New York: McGraw-Hill, 1994.

Hilton-Jones D, Squier M, Taylor D, Matthews P (eds). *Metabolic Myopathies*. London: WB Saunders, 1995.

Karpati G, Hilton-Jones D, Griggs R (eds), *Disorders of Voluntary Muscle*, 7th edn. Cambridge: Cambridge University Press, 2001.

Lane RJM. *Handbook of Muscle Disease*. New York: Marcel Dekker, 1996.

Specific diseases

Acid maltase deficiency

Kikuchi T, Yang HW, Pennybacker M et al. Clinical and metabolic correction of Pompe disease by enzyme therapy in acid maltase-deficient quail. *J Clin Invest* 1998; 101: 827–833.

Myophosphorylase deficiency

el-Schahawi M, Tsujino S, Shanske S, DiMauro S. Diagnosis of McArdle's disease by molecular genetic analysis of blood. *Neurology* 1996; 47: 579–580.

Debrancher enzyme deficiency

Coleman RA, Winter HS, Wolf B, Gilchrist JM, Chen YT. Glycogen storage disease type III (glycogen debranching enzyme deficiency): correlation of biochemical defects with myopathy and cardiomyopathy. *Ann Int Med* 1992; 116: 896–900.

Phosphofructokinase deficiency

Raben N & Sherman JB. Mutations in muscle phosphofructokinase gene. *Hum Mutat* 1995; 6: 1–6.

chapter 9

Toxic and endocrine myopathies

The conditions discussed in this chapter are arguably the most frequently encountered acquired myopathies in clinical practice. If the offending toxin is removed, or the underlying endocrine disorder is corrected, then recovery is usual. Somewhat paradoxically, they are encountered relatively infrequently in specialist muscle clinics because, more often than not, the underlying condition was evident before the myopathy developed and the patient was already under suitably experienced medical supervision. With the endocrine myopathies (Figure 9.1) weakness is often just one part, and sometimes only a small one, of a multisystem disorder

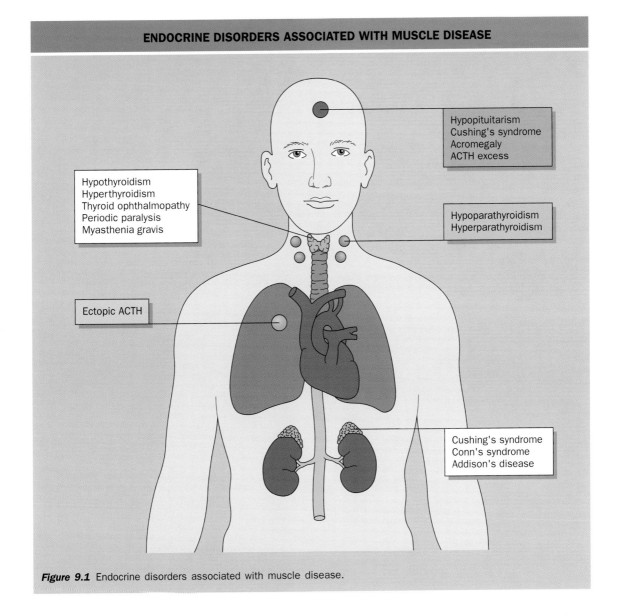

ENDOCRINE DISORDERS ASSOCIATED WITH MUSCLE DISEASE

Hypopituitarism
Cushing's syndrome
Acromegaly
ACTH excess

Hypothyroidism
Hyperthyroidism
Thyroid ophthalmopathy
Periodic paralysis
Myasthenia gravis

Hypoparathyroidism
Hyperparathyroidism

Ectopic ACTH

Cushing's syndrome
Conn's syndrome
Addison's disease

Figure 9.1 Endocrine disorders associated with muscle disease.

and the additional features readily point to the correct diagnosis. Myopathy is an under-recognised feature of chronic alcoholism, ignored because of the many other physical consequences of the condition. In nearly all of the conditions to be discussed the muscle pathology and neurophysiological findings are non-specific and diagnosis is based on clinical evaluation and metabolic/endocrine studies.

Drug-induced myopathies

A wise dictum is to assume that your patient's ills are due to the drugs and toxins (licit and otherwise) that they are taking, until proved otherwise. This is illustrated by a recent case report in a respected medical journal, which will not be cited to avoid embarrassment to the authors; a patient presenting with generalised weakness underwent extensive investigations, including neurophysiological studies and muscle biopsy, before it was appreciated that the cause was profound hypokalaemia secondary to diuretic treatment for hypertension!

In general, the precise mechanisms of drug-induced myotoxicity are poorly understood. Furthermore, some drugs are neurotoxic as well as myotoxic. In practice, the most useful approach to classification is to use a combination of clinical features and pathological changes. Table 9.1 summarises the major forms of drug-induced myopathy and lists some of the more commonly implicated drugs. Several drugs may have more than one form of presentation.

Focal myopathy reflects local muscle fibre damage and fibrosis following intramuscular injections. The mildest form is reflected in elevation of the serum creatine kinase following such injections (and perhaps also after muscle sampling during needle electromyography). Repeated injections may cause extensive fibrosis and contracture and may be seen in illicit drug-abusers (e.g. with pethidine or pentazocine).

Painful myopathy may take the form of isolated myalgia, myalgia with weakness, or a more severe syndrome with extensive myonecrosis – the latter overlaps with acute rhabdomyolysis. Amongst the most commonly implicated drugs are the cholesterol-lowering agents (e.g. clofibrate, gemfibrozil, and the HMG-CoA reductase inhibitors, which are often referred to as statins). The risk of myopathy is significantly increased by a number of factors; combined use of two cholesterol-lowering agents, concomitant use of cyclosporin, renal failure, nephrotic syndrome, and hypothyroidism. Myopathy is common with emetine use and may be

Table 9.1 *Drug-induced myopathies*

Focal myopathy	Intramuscular injections
Acute/subacute painful myopathy	Amiodarone
	β-blockers
	Cholesterol-lowering agents
	Ciclosporin
	Emetine
	ε-aminocaproic acid
	Opiates
	Vincristine
	Zidovudine
Acute rhabdomyolysis	Amphetamines
	Cocaine
	Opiates
	Phencyclidine
Chronic painless myopathy	Amiodarone
	Chloroquine
	Colchicine
	Corticosteroids
	Perhexiline
Hypokalaemia	Amphotericin B
	Carbenoxolone
	Diuretics
	Liquorice
	Purgatives
Inflammatory myopathy	D-penicillamine
	Procainamide
Myasthenic syndrome	Antibiotics (typically aminoglycosides)
	D-penicillamine

fatal, particularly if there is an associated cardiomyopathy. Increasingly prevalent is zidovudine myopathy; myalgia is a feature in about one in ten patients but some then go on to develop generalised weakness, typically one year or more after starting treatment. The drug inhibits mitochondrial DNA polymerase and the myopathy is associated with reduced levels of mitochondrial DNA and ragged-red fibres, as well as with inflammatory changes. Partial or complete recovery follows drug withdrawal. Vincristine has neurotoxic and myotoxic effects, the latter manifesting as a painful proximal necrotizing myopathy associated with autophagic destruction of fibres.

Acute rhabdomyolysis represents a more severe continuation of the above. It is seen most frequently in the setting of drug-abuse and has parallels with acute alcoholic myopathy, discussed below.

Chronic painless myopathy is the least dramatic, but at the same time the commonest, form of drug-induced myopathy. Iatrogenic corticosteroid myopathy is the most important and the clinical features are similar to those of Cushing's syndrome (see below). Muscle discomfort may be a feature, but severe pain is absent. Mild cases are certainly often overlooked. Myopathy is more likely to develop with the fluorinated corticosteroids (e.g. dexamethasone, betamethasone and triamcinolone) and may complicate topical as well as systemic usage. The serum creatine kinase is normal, electromyography shows myopathic features, and histology show type II (particularly IIb) muscle fibre atrophy. Recovery follows drug withdrawal and during treatment the myopathic effects can be ameliorated by regular exercise. A particularly dramatic syndrome is that of an acute myopathy precipitated by high-dose parenteral corticosteroids often, but not always, given in combination with a neuromuscular blocking agent. This was first noted in patients being treated for asthma but has now been reported in other settings, including the treatment of myasthenic crisis. Weakness may be profound, and accompanied by respiratory failure. Recovery occurs over 6–12 months. Pathologically there are small angular fibres and an extraordinary selective loss of myosin filaments. Chloroquine is associated with a potentially severe vacuolar myopathy, sometimes complicated by a cardiomyopathy. Slow recovery follows drug withdrawal.

Hypokalaemia causes generalised weakness (so-called secondary periodic paralysis if the weakness is episodic) that may be painful and is associated with elevation of the serum creatine kinase and sometimes with myoglobinuria. The respiratory muscle may be involved. The commonest causes are therapeutic use of diuretics and abuse of liquorice and purgatives.

Inflammatory myopathy secondary to drugs is relatively uncommon but may be seen in zidovudine myopathy (see above), with D-penicillamine, and as part of a lupus-like syndrome associated with procainamide therapy.

Myasthenic syndromes have been reported with a number of drugs, notably aminoglycoside antibiotics and β-blockers, but it may well be that in many instances the drug exposed sub-clinical myasthenia. In such cases presentation is early, in distinction to the myasthenic disorder induced by D-penicillamine which is mediated by immune mechanisms and which presents months or years after initiating therapy.

Table 9.2 *Toxin-induced myopathies*

Ethanol
    Acute alcoholic myopathy
    Chronic alcoholic myopathy
Dietary
    Eosinophilia-myalgia syndrome
    Toxic oil syndrome
    Germanium
    Vitamin E
Animal toxins (venoms)
Organophosphorus insecticides

Toxic myopathies

To distinguish between toxin-induced and drug-induced myopathies is rather artificial, and some might argue that ethanol is a useful therapeutic agent! Table 9.2 lists what might be called "non-prescribed" causes of myotoxicity.

Ethanol causes two forms of myopathy. Chronic alcoholic myopathy is by far the commonest and is certainly under-recognised. Probably two-thirds of chronic alcoholics have clinical evidence of myopathy, although distinguishing from the general effects of malnutrition and from the likely co-existent neuropathy may be difficult. Indeed, some authors have questioned whether there is much in the way of a direct toxic effect on muscle, arguing that the weakness is mainly neuropathic in origin. The clinical picture is that of painless, relatively mild, proximal weakness affecting the pelvic more than the shoulder-girdle musculature. Acute alcoholic myopathy is a rarer but more dramatic affair. It typically develops in a chronic alcoholic following a binge. The problem may be generalised or restricted to one or a few muscles. Typically pain and cramping precedes the onset of weakness, which is accompanied by muscle swelling, but occasionally weakness develops without pain. Lower limb involvement may be misdiagnosed as deep venous thrombosis. Swelling may induce a compartment syndrome. There is extensive muscle fibre breakdown (rhabdomyolysis) with gross elevation of the serum creatine kinase, and myoglobinuria which poses a risk to renal function. Hyperkalaemia may be marked, particularly in the presence of renal failure. Recovery, which may be incomplete, occurs over several weeks.

Dietary contaminants and dietary fads may lead to myopathy. Although now primarily of historical interest, the eosinophilia-myalgia and Spanish toxic oil syndromes illustrate vividly the potential for mass poisoning. The eosinophilia-myalgia syndrome was caused by a contaminant in a batch of L-tryptophan made by a single manufacturer. Symptoms included myalgia, skin rash, dyspnoea, arthralgia, fever and weight loss, with later a scleroderma-like skin infiltration. Some patients had persistent weakness. Similar clinical features were seen in the Spanish toxic oil syndrome, caused by ingestion of an illegally imported, reprocessed, denatured rapeseed oil. Germanium intoxication causes weakness, renal failure and, sometimes, death. The weakness is associated with a vacuolar myopathy and some evidence that mitochondrial function is disturbed. Vitamin E excess has been reported to cause a proximal necrotizing myopathy.

Animal toxins may be myotoxic, the best-known examples being snake venoms. Polymyositis has been reported complicating poisoning by ciguatera, a toxin originating from a coral reef organism which man then ingests in seafood.

Organophosphorus insecticides irreversibly inhibit cholinesterases and cause generalised weakness, including respiratory failure. Given adequate supportive measures, recovery occurs within 10–14 days. In some patients, and in experimental models, necrotizing myopathy has been described.

Thyroid disorders

Myopathy is a feature of both hypo- and hyperthyroidism. Thyroid ophthalmopathy is an autoimmune disorder in which the patient may be euthyroid. There is an increased incidence of thyroid disease in patients with myasthenia gravis, and vice versa, and thyroid dysfunction can exacerbate myasthenic weakness.

Hypothyroidism
Proximal weakness can be demonstrated in most patients, but is rarely the presenting problem. Myopathic symptoms are present in over 80% of patients, and apart from weakness include myalgia, stiffness and cramps. The most characteristic finding on examination is delayed relaxation of the tendon reflexes (most easily seen at the ankle or the brachioradialis/supinator reflex). Myoedema and muscle hypertrophy are rarer findings. The combination of substantial muscle hypertrophy, weakness and slowness of movement is sometimes referred to as the Kocher-Debré-Semelaigne syndrome in childhood (with

congenital hypothyroidism), or Hoffman's syndrome in adults (in whom painful cramps may also occur), but it is unlikely that either is a specific entity and they reflect simply severe hypothyroid myopathy.

The serum creatine kinase is elevated in about 90% of patients with hypothyroidism, even in the absence of demonstrable weakness. Indeed, subclinical hypothyroidism is one of the commonest causes of apparently unexplained hyperCKaemia (i.e. a raised serum creatine kinase in the absence of overt muscle disease). Electromyographic abnormalities are seen in many, but not all, cases but are non-specific. Complex repetitive discharges are present in up to one-third, but myotonia is not a feature. Similarly, muscle biopsy findings are non-specific, typically with type II fibre atrophy.

Full recovery of the myopathy occurs, but may take several months, once the patient is rendered euthyroid.

Hyperthyroidism
Fewer than 10% of patients present because of weakness, but about one-half have weakness as a symptom and over 80% have demonstrable weakness. The weakness is typically proximal and somewhat different to other limb-girdle syndromes because the shoulder muscles may be more affected than those of the pelvic girdle. In up to one-fifth there may be significant distal weakness. Prominent bulbar weakness occasionally occurs.

Paradoxically, although the weakness in thyrotoxic myopathy is usually more striking than in hypothyroid myopathy, the serum creatine kinase is usually normal. As in hypothyroid myopathy electromyographic and muscle biopsy findings are non-specific and do not contribute greatly towards the diagnosis.

Full recovery occurs within months of successful treatment of the hyperthyroidism, by whatever method.

Thyroid ophthalmopathy
Graves described eye involvement in association with hyperthyroidism, but it may also occur in euthyroid and hypothyroid individuals. It is an autoimmune disorder for which the afferent and efferent limbs are not yet fully understood. Thyroid-stimulating immunoglobulins are detectable in over 90% of patients with Graves' disease and in about one-half of euthyroid patients with ophthalmopathy.

Eyelid lag and retraction are common in thyrotoxicosis. The next stage of the ophthalmopathy is itching, redness of the conjunctivae and eyelid swelling. Subsequently the extraocular muscles and orbital soft tissues swell, causing diplopia and proptosis. Corneal

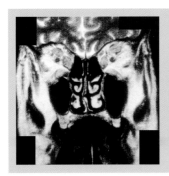

Figure 9.2 Thyroid ophthalmopathy. Coronal MRI scan, through the level of the orbits, shows extraocular muscle hypertrophy. (Courtesy of Dr P. Anslow.)

ulceration may develop and vision deteriorates due to the development of papilloedema and optic nerve compression. All of the changes described can be unilateral. An important subgroup, particularly for neurologists, is those patients who present with diplopia only, without the other suggestive features pointing towards thyroid dysfunction.

The diagnosis is easy if typical clinical features are associated with abnormal biochemistry. If the thyroxine (T4), tri-iodothyronine (T3) and thyroid-stimulating (TSH) levels are normal, then the next stage of investigation includes a thyrotrophin-releasing hormone (TRH) stimulation test and assay of antithyroglobulin and antimicrosomal antibodies.

Orbital imaging (ultrasound, CT or MRI) can show the characteristic extraocular muscle swelling and may be very helpful when laboratory support for the diagnosis is lacking (Figure 9.2).

Hyper- or hypo-thyroidism should be treated but this does not always improve the ophthalmopathy, and of course some patients are euthyroid at presentation. Eyelid lag and retraction may respond to topical 10% guanethidine. If major problems persist treatment options include surgical decompression, high-dose prednisolone, and orbital irradiation. Surgery offers the quickest response if sight is threatened. Lateral tarsorrhaphy may help to protect the cornea.

Periodic paralysis

The clinical features of thyrotoxic periodic paralysis (TPP) closely parallel those of primary hypokalaemic periodic paralysis (hypoPP) and are discussed in Chapter 6. TPP differs from hypoPP in the following ways; it is rarely familial, there is an even greater male predominance, the incidence and prevalence is enormously greater in Orientals, onset is typically later (in adult life), and administration of thyroid hormone precipitates attacks in patients with TPP but not in those with hypoPP.

All forms of hyperthyroidism have been associated with TPP, but Graves' disease is by far the commonest. The serum potassium level may fall somewhat during an attack. Electromyography and muscle biopsy between attacks are typically normal.

Oral potassium may speed recovery from an attack and propranolol may prevent attacks, but the main aim is to make the patient euthyroid, after which the attacks will cease.

Myasthenia gravis and thyroid disease

Hyperthyroidism and hypothyroidism each occur in about 5% of patients with myasthenia gravis (MG). Up to one-third of patients with MG have thyroid autoantibodies and in one pathological series nearly one in five patients had histological evidence of Hashimoto's thyroiditis. Conversely, the prevalence of MG in patients with thyrotoxicosis is about 30 times greater than in the general population, although only about 0.1% of thyrotoxic patients will develop MG. Thyrotoxicosis may precede or follow the onset of MG. Myasthenic symptoms are typically exacerbated by thyrotoxicosis.

Disorders of the pituitary–adrenal axis

Although myopathy may be seen in several disorders of the pituitary-adrenal axis, by far and away the commonest, and also generally the most severe, is glucocorticoid excess and because of the clinical similarities it is appropriate to consider Cushing's syndrome and iatrogenic corticosteroid excess together.

Hypopituitarism

Panhypopituitarism is associated with generalized weakness and fatigue, which probably relate mainly to deficiency of thyroid and adrenal cortical hormones. These symptoms improve with appropriate replacement therapy. In isolated growth hormone deficiency in childhood there is impaired muscle development, but as it parallels the general failure of growth weakness is not usually a feature.

Acromegaly

Growth hormone (GH) excess is usually due to a functioning pituitary adenoma, rarely to production from a tumour elsewhere. About one-half of patients have evidence of myopathy with symptoms including proximal weakness, fatigue, and myalgia. There is little muscle wasting.

The serum creatine kinase is normal or mildly elevated and as in so many endocrine myopathies EMG and muscle biopsy show non-specific features only.

Treatment may be by surgery or irradiation. If these are not possible, or if after such treatment GH levels remain elevated, the somatostatin analogue octreotide may be of value. There is some evidence that weakness may persist even if GH levels are returned to normal.

Adrenocorticotrophin excess

Adrenocorticotrophin (ACTH) excess due to a functioning pituitary adenoma or from ectopic production from a tumour elsewhere is associated with high glucocorticoid levels. Myopathy in these circumstances is usually attributed to the glucocorticoid excess. In Nelson's syndrome, following adrenalectomy, there is a high level of ACTH in the absence of raised glucocorticoid levels and myopathy has been reported, although it is probably uncommon and mild.

Cushing's syndrome

The myopathy of Cushing's syndrome is believed to be due to glucocorticoid excess and as the clinical and laboratory features closely parallel iatrogenic corticosteroid myopathy they are usually considered together.

Cushing's syndrome may be due to an ACTH-producing pituitary adenoma (about two-thirds of cases), to a tumour of the adrenal cortex (one-sixth), or to ectopic production from a tumour (usually bronchial) elsewhere (one-sixth). Pituitary Cushing's is commoner in women, ectopic Cushing's in men, and adrenal Cushing's in children. Weakness is present in some 60% of patients with Cushing's syndrome and is an important feature distinguishing it from other conditions that cause obesity and hirsutes.

Iatrogenic corticosteroid myopathy can be caused by any of the currently available glucocorticoid drugs but is most likely to be seen in association with the 9α fluorinated steroids; dexamethasone, betamethasone and triamcinolone. Myopathy may even occur with topical use (e.g. betamethasone).

The clinical picture is of proximal weakness, typically involving the pelvic girdle musculature before the shoulder girdle, often accompanied by myalgia. Bulbar and respiratory muscle involvement is rare.

The serum creatine kinase is usually normal, as is EMG. Muscle biopsy findings are non-specific but the most consistent finding is type II fibre atrophy affecting the IIb fibres before the IIa fibres.

Corticosteroid drugs have a major role in the treatment of the idiopathic inflammatory myopathies (and

Table 9.3 Distinguishing between weakness due to myositis and that due to corticosteroid-induced myopathy.

	Findings in favour of weakness being due to:	
	Myositis	Corticosteroid myopathy
Serum CK markedly raised	++	−
Inflammation in muscle biopsy	+++	−
EMG fibrillation potentials	+	−
No other signs of steroid excess	+	−
Creatinuria and elevated CK	+	−
Type II fibre atrophy & no inflammation	−	+
Greater weakness shortly after Increase in steroid dose	−	+
Increased serum LDH and normal CK	−	+
Creatinuria and normal CK	−	+

CK = creatine kinase
LDH = lactate dehydrogenase

also myasthenic syndromes) and it may occasionally be difficult to determine whether deterioration in strength when on treatment is due to reactivation of the underlying disorder (which would necessitate an increase in drug dosage), or to the development of a corticosteroid myopathy (when dose reduction would be indicated). Factors favouring reactivation of myositis or steroid myopathy are summarised in Table 9.3. If uncertainty remains the corticosteroid dose should be lowered and the clinical and laboratory response observed.

When Cushing's syndrome is successfully treated the myopathy resolves, as indeed it does when corticosteroids are withdrawn in the case of iatrogenic corticosteroid myopathy. If steroid drug treatment must continue then the lowest possible dose should be used, a non-fluorinated compound such as prednisolone is to be preferred, and an alternate-day regimen instituted if satisfactory for controlling the primary disease process.

Addison's disease

This is usually an autoimmune disorder, less common causes including adrenoleucodystrophy, tuberculosis, secondary tumour, amyloidosis and granulomatous diseases. Generalized weakness, fatigue and myalgia are present in up to one-half of patients, and respond to glucocorticoid replacement. Rarely, secondary hyperkalaemic periodic paralysis develops.

The serum creatine kinase is normal or mildly elevated and EMG normal. There have been few reports detailing muscle biopsy findings.

The diagnosis of Addison's disease is established either by simultaneous assay of plasma ACTH and cortisol, or by a tetracosactrin stimulation test.

Conn's syndrome

Primary aldosteronism causes hypokalaemia, which in turn may cause weakness. Initiation of diuretic therapy may precipitate severe weakness and may be the first pointer to the diagnosis, which is established by demonstration of elevated plasma or urine aldosterone levels and depressed plasma renin activity.

Metabolic bone disease

This broad term is useful when considering the myopathic disorders associated with vitamin D deficiency (osteomalacia), parathyroid dysfunction, and renal disease.

Vitamin D_3 is synthesized in the skin, under the influence of ultraviolet light, from provitamin D. It is transported to the liver, where it undergoes 25-hydroxylation, and then to the kidney where it is further hydroxylated to either 1,25- or 24,25-dihydroxy vitamin D. The 1,25 form is the more active and its synthesis is stimulated by low levels of serum calcium and phosphate and by parathyroid hormone (PTH). PTH secretion is stimulated by hypocalcaemia. 1,25-dihydroxy vitamin D promotes intestinal calcium absorption, bone resorption, and renal reabsorption of phosphate. PTH directly increases intestinal absorption and renal reabsorption of calcium and increases bone resorption, as well as promoting 1,25-dihydroxyvitamin D production. The intimate relationships between calcium, vitamin D and PTH can readily be appreciated.

Osteomalacia

This may be due to dietary deficiency or malabsorption, or be secondary to renal disease. One of the most constant features is bone pain, most prominent in the pelvis, femora and ribs. It has been suggested that pain, limitation of movement leading to disuse atrophy, and general effects of malnutrition are the main causes of weakness, but there is good evidence to suggest that there is a true primary myopathy. The pelvic girdle musculature is most involved and is associated with a waddling gait and Gower's manoeuvre. In about one-third of patients weakness is the presenting symptom. Muscle pain may be present but is less intense than the bone pain.

The diagnosis of osteomalacia depends upon bone densitometry, and demonstration of low blood calcium and phosphate levels with elevation of alkaline phosphatase activity. EMG and muscle biopsy show only non-specific changes and the serum creatine kinase is typically normal.

Oral vitamin D is effective for treating dietary deficiency and malabsorption (higher doses being needed), but in renal disease the preferred treatment is 1-α-hydroxycholecalciferol which does not require the renal hydroxylation step to be activated.

Bone pain responds rapidly with treatment but weakness takes longer to resolve.

Renal and dialysis osteodystrophy

Renal osteodystrophy describes the combination of disturbed vitamin D metabolism and secondary hyperparathyroidism that invariably complicate chronic uraemia. End-stage renal failure is often accompanied by pelvic girdle weakness, sometimes with buttock and thigh pain. Improvement follows dialysis, renal transplantation, and treatment with vitamin D or its analogues.

Dialysis osteodystrophy was probably due to aluminium toxicity, from high aluminium levels in the tap water used to prepare the dialysate and from aluminium-containing antacids. Features included severe myopathy, bone pain and fractures.

Parathyroid disease

Primary hyperparathyroidism is caused by a functioning parathyroid adenoma and is associated with high serum levels of PTH. Severe hyperparathyroidism may cause weakness but is now rarely reported, perhaps in part because the widespread use of biochemical autoanalysers, which include "routine" calcium estimations, has led to earlier diagnosis and treatment.

Hypoparathyroidism is usually secondary to surgical removal of the parathyroid glands. The only common neuromuscular feature of hypoparathyroidism is tetany secondary to hypocalcaemia. Myopathy has been reported rarely in hypoparathyroidism and pseudohypoparathyroidism and even when present is mild.

Secondary hyperparathyroidism, as noted above, is common when there is any disturbance of vitamin D metabolism.

Selected further reading

Textbooks and reviews

Argov Z, Ruff R. Toxic and iatrogenic myopathies. In: Karpati G, Hilton-Jones D, Griggs R (eds). *Disorders of Voluntary Muscle* 7th edn. Cambridge: Cambridge University Press, 2001.

Hilton-Jones D, Squier M, Taylor D, Matthews P (eds). *Metabolic Myopathies*. London: WB Saunders, 1995.

Victor M & Sieb JP. Myopathies due to drugs, toxins, and nutritional deficiency. In: Engel AG, Franzini-Armstrong C (eds). *Myology* 2nd edn. New York: McGraw-Hill, 1994.

Kaminsky HJ & Ruff RL. (1994) Endocrine Myopathies. In: Engel AG, Franzini-Armstrong C (eds). *Myology* 2nd edn. New York: McGraw-Hill, 1994: 1726–1753.

Specific diseases
Alcoholic myopathy

Estruch R, Sacanella E, Fernandez-Sola J et al. Natural history of alcoholic myopathy: a 5-year study. *Alcohol Clin Exp Res* 1998; 22: 2023–2028.

Dysthyroid myopathy

Weetman AP & Wiersinga WM. Current management of thyroid-associated ophthalmopathy in Europe. Results of an international survey. *Clin Endocrinol Oxf* 1998; 49: 21–28.

Papadopoulos KI, Diep T, Cleland B, Lunn NW. Thyrotoxic periodic paralysis: report of three cases and review of the literature. *J Int Med* 1997; 241: 521–524.

Pituitary-adrenal axis disorders

Fischer JR, Baer RK. Acute myopathy associated with combined use of corticosteroids and neuromuscular blocking agents. *Ann Pharmacother* 1996; 30: 1437–1445.

Myopathy and metabolic bone disease

Burn DJ, Bates D. Neurology and the kidney. *J Neurol Neurosurg Psych* 1998; 65: 810–821.

Reginato AJ, Falasca GF, Pappu R, McKnight B, Agha A. Musculoskeletal manifestations of osteomalacia: report of 26 cases and literature review. *Semin Arthritis Rheum* 1999; 28: 287–304.

chapter 10

Miscellaneous muscle disorders

Tumours of skeletal muscle

Primary tumours of skeletal muscle are uncommon and their classification is not entirely satisfactory. Their importance lies in part in the differential of other conditions including focal myositis, pyogenic abscesses, tendon rupture and muscle herniation through fascia. With the notable exception of local spread into pectoral muscles from breast carcinoma, secondary tumours are perhaps surprisingly rare, given that muscle is highly vascular and accounts for up to 40% of body weight. Evidence of tumour emboli in skeletal muscle may be not that uncommon pathologically but is rarely identified clinically. Tumours of supporting tissues are also rare and include dermoid tumours and angiomata.

Rhabdomyomas in adults tend to develop in the head, neck and throat region. Cardiac rhabdomyomas in childhood may be associated with tuberous sclerosis. Embryonal rhabdomyomas in early childhood affect the head and neck region, and also the genitourinary tract where the grape-like appearance gives rise to the term sarcoma botryoides. Alveolar rhabdomyomas in older children are aggressive tumours that metastasise and have a poor prognosis. Similarly, pleomorphic rhabdomyosarcomas in adults, which tend to arise in the legs, metastasise early.

Paraneoplastic syndromes

If metabolic and endocrine disorders are included there are many paraneoplastic myopathies (Table 10.1). This Table excludes paraneoplastic disorders of neuromuscular transmission. In over one-half of patients with Lambert-Eaton myasthenic syndrome there is an underlying neoplasm, and of those some 80% are small-cell lung cancers. In myasthenia gravis, a thymoma is present in about 10% of patients. Myasthenic syndromes and endocrine and metabolic disorders are discussed in Chapters 9 and 12.

Table 10.1 *Paraneoplastic myopathies*

Dermatomyositis

Carcinomatous neuromyopathy

Acute necrotising myopathy

Metabolic
- Hypokalaemia
    - Conn's syndrome
    - Renin-secreting tumours
    - Cushing's syndrome
    - Acute leukaemia
    - Rectal villous adenoma
    - Hyperkalaemia
    - Addison's disease due to tumour destruction of glands
    - Hypercalcaemia
    - Parathyroid hormone secreting tumours
    - Bone metastases
    - Myeloma

Endocrine
- Hypopituitarism
    - Adenoma
    - Craniopharyngioma
    - Secondary pituitary tumour
- ACTH excess
    - Ectopic tumour production
- Growth hormone excess
    - Pituitary adenoma
- Glucocorticoid excess
    - Pituitary adenoma
    - Adrenal adenoma
    - Ectopic ACTH production
- Hypoadrenalism
    - Addison's disease due to tumour destruction of glands
- Thyroxine excess
    - Functional thyroid tumour
- Parathyroid hormone (PTH) excess
    - Parathyroid adenoma
    - Ectopic PTH production

Carcinomatous neuromyopathy

Although one of the most frequently invoked causes of weakness in association with carcinoma it is a poorly defined entity. It is used to describe a syndrome of proximal weakness and wasting which can run a subacute or chronic course and in which the tendon reflexes are often depressed. It is probable that many such cases are predominantly neuropathic in origin.

Acute necrotizing myopathy

This condition probably overlaps with dermatomyositis but the term has been used to describe a syndrome of rapid progression of generalised weakness in which muscle biopsy shows a non-inflammatory necrotizing myopathy.

Dermatomyositis

The clinical details of this condition are discussed in Chapter 5. The older literature with respect to association with tumour is unsatisfactory, because of failure to differentiate accurately between dermatomyositis and polymyositis. About 20% of patients with dermatomyositis have an underlying malignancy and sometimes the development of dermatomyositis heralds reappearance of a previously treated tumour (Figure 10.1). An associated neoplasm is rare in childhood and commoner in older patients. Thus, in an adult presenting with dermatomyositis there is an obligation to search for a tumour. There is no link with any particular tumour type, as there is for Lambert-Eaton myasthenic syndrome, and so investigations have to be broad; general physical examination, breast, rectal and vaginal examination, blood tests, chest X-ray, and often a scan of the abdomen. More detailed investigations might be indicated by the history; e.g. cross-sectional chest scanning in a smoker, endoscopy if gastrointestinal symptoms are present. If there is a link between cancer and polymyositis, which remains debatable, it is substantially weaker than with dermatomyositis.

Chronic fatigue syndrome

Although a small part of the voluminous literature concerning chronic fatigue syndrome (CFS) is of high quality, much of it is outrageously bad and includes frequent cross-referencing and reduplication of unsubstantiated claims. Despite this, a picture is beginning to emerge. Neuromuscular symptoms include fatigue and myalgia, and often a perception of weakness, but these are often overshadowed by central symptoms such as impaired memory and concentration, sleep disturbance

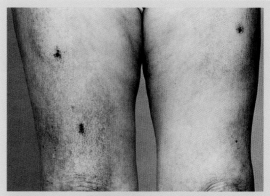
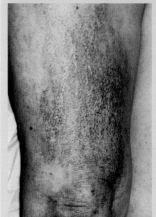

Figure 10.1
Dermatomyositis. The patient had previously been treated for a colonic carcinoma. The development several years later of dermatomyositis was rapidly followed by the identification of tumour recurrence.

and emotional lability. That the syndrome exists is undoubted: it is difficult to find any literature suggesting that it does not even though patient support groups frequently say that many doctors deny its existence. It is clearly a syndrome, in that it is of diverse aetiology. In the majority of patients no evidence of physical disease can be found and psychological factors seem readily evident. Patients with a range of "classical" neurological conditions, including several neuromuscular disorders (particularly myasthenia gravis), are not infrequently misdiagnosed as having CFS and it is arguably the neurologists main role to exclude such conditions.

In a few patients the myopathic symptoms might be due to an underlying metabolic myopathy, in which case any additional non-myopathic symptomatology including apparently psychiatric symptoms, is presumably secondary. However, the number of patients in whom a specific enzyme defect, such as myophosphorylase deficiency, is identified is vanishingly small. Abnormalities demonstrated by magnetic resonance spectroscopy, and of lactate generation during aerobic exercise, are of dubious significance and may at least in part be attributable to deconditioning due to lack of exercise.

No convincing muscle histological changes have been demonstrated, traditional biochemical assays of intermediary energy pathways reveal no abnormality, and reports of persistent enteroviral infection of muscle are of dubious significance. Physiological studies looking at activation, twitch properties, endurance, and recovery have shown no abnormality.

In summary, no evidence exists for primary neuromuscular involvement in the vast majority of patients with CFS.

Myositis ossificans

This term is used to describe two unrelated conditions. Despite the name, they are not primarily inflammatory disorders. Localized myositis ossificans usually arises as a result of trauma, either minor repeated trauma (for example, in sportsmen or women) or a single substantial injury. Initially there is localized swelling and tenderness, which is followed by bone formation. Small lesions may resolve spontaneously but larger areas of calcification may need to be resected. Fibrodysplasia ossificans progressiva is inherited as an autosomal dominant, but the genetic defect is unknown. Shortening of the great toe, less frequently the thumb, is present almost invariably. Endochondral ossification of skeletal muscles occurs in a specific order and the patients are described as developing a second skeleton. It causes profound immobility and patients become wheelchair-bound by the third decade of life. No treatment is available.

Compartment syndromes

Some muscles are contained within semi-rigid fibro-osseous compartments, the most important examples being the anterior tibial compartment and the volar compartment of the forearm. If the muscles within these compartments swell the pressure rises rapidly (a situation similar to rising intracranial pressure, because the brain is also contained within a rigid compartment). The most important cause of swelling is ischaemia due to arterial problems (e.g. compression due to displaced fracture, tourniquet pressure, clamping during surgery, haematoma) or direct trauma. Acute alcoholic myopathy is another cause. The rising pressure further impedes capillary blood flow and thus a vicious circle of increasing ischaemia develops. Nerves within the compartment become ischaemic and if the pressure is high enough for long enough infarction may occur.

The major clinical features are pain, swelling, and sensory and motor involvement relating to the peripheral nerves compressed within the compartment, but of course not all of these features will be evident in the unconscious patient. Extensive muscle necrosis may lead to myoglobinuria and renal failure (crush syndrome). Compartment pressure can be measured using a wick-catheter. Treatment is by subcutaneous fasciotomy. Permanent muscle contracture secondary to fibrosis of the damaged muscle is known as Volkmann's ischaemic contracture.

Chronic involvement of the tibial compartment is recognised, particularly in athletes. Local pain develops on exercise and resolves with rest. Symptoms parallel an increase in pressure within the compartment during exercise, as can be demonstrated by wick-catheter studies. The problem may resolve after a period of prolonged rest but in some cases fasciotomy is required.

Selected further reading

Tumours of skeletal muscle
Newton WA, Gehan EA, Webber BL et al. Classification of rhabdomyosarcomas and related sarcomas. Pathologic aspects and proposal for a new classification – an Intergroup Rhabdomyosarcoma Study. *Cancer* 1995; 76: 1073–1085.

Paraneoplastic myopathies
Hilton-Jones D. The clinical features of some miscellaneous neuromuscular disorders. In: Walton JN, Karpati G, Hilton-Jones D (eds). *Disorders of Voluntary Muscle* 6th edn. Edinburgh: Churchill Livingstone, Edinburgh, 1994: 967–987.

Chronic fatigue syndrome
Hilton-Jones D. The clinical features of some miscellaneous neuromuscular disorders. In: Walton JN, Karpati G, Hilton-Jones D (eds).

Disorders of Voluntary Muscle 6th edn. Edinburgh: Churchill Livingstone, 1999: 967–987.
Wessely S, Nimnuan C, Sharpe M. Functional somatic syndromes: one or many? *Lancet* 1999; 354: 936–939.

Fibrodysplasia ossificans progressiva
Kaplan FS, Delatycki M, Gannon FH et al. Fibrodysplasia ossificans progressiva. In: Emery AEH (ed) *Neuromuscular Disorders: clinical and molecular genetics*. Chichester: John Wiley & Sons, 1998: 289–321.

Compartment syndromes
Trice M, Colwell CW. A historical review of compartment syndrome and Volkmann's ischemic contracture. *Hand Clin* 1998; 14: 335–341.

chapter 11

Congenital myopathies

The disorders to be discussed in this section present a number of difficulties with respect to nomenclature and classification, although this is slowly being resolved as their genetic and molecular bases are being unravelled. The term congenital is a problem in itself, for some of these conditions are not evident at birth and occasionally are not diagnosed until adult life. However, typical clinicopathological features include presentation as a "floppy infant", morphological changes such as high-arched palate, long face and skeletal deformity, generalised muscle slimness and weakness, little or no progression, normal or only slightly elevated serum creatine kinase, and specific structural changes within muscle (indeed, they are sometimes called ultrastructural myopathies). The disorders may be sporadic, or show autosomal recessive, dominant, or X-linked inheritance, and some disorders show more than one pattern of inheritance.

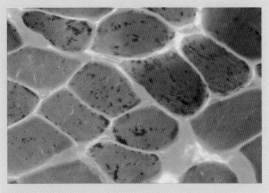

Figure 11.1 Nemaline myopathy. Modified Gomori trichrome stain.

dominant form have recently been identified – alpha-tropomyosin (*TPM3*) and alpha actin (*ACTA1*), as has the gene for the commoner recessive form (the nebulin gene).

Nemaline myopathy

Most cases present at birth as floppy infants, but later onset can occur. There is facial and proximal limb weakness. Dysmorphic features (long face, high-arched palate, chest deformity) are common and, as in the other congenital myopathies, reflect intra-uterine and congenital weakness. Respiratory failure, probably indicating diaphragmatic involvement, is relatively common and respiratory function must be monitored throughout life. It can be managed by nocturnal mask positive pressure assisted ventilation. Typically, progression of weakness is very slow.

The major pathological feature of this condition is the presence of nemaline rods in the subsarcolemmal region (Figure 11.1) – these appear red using the Gomori trichrome method. They are derived from the Z-bands. They are not pathognomonic in that they may be seen as a secondary phenomenon in other disorders.

Nemaline myopathy may be inherited as an autosomal dominant or recessive. Two genes for the rarer

Central core disease (CCD)

This was the first described of the conditions later to be called the congenital myopathies. It has an important association with malignant hyperthermia (MH). Presentation is typically in infancy, as a floppy baby or with delayed motor milestones, but asymptomatic adult cases are also recognised (and are often discovered during family screening studies following the identification of an affected individual with either myopathy or MH). The weakness is usually mild and is either generalised, also involving the face, or affects mainly proximal lower limb muscles. Scoliosis, foot deformities, congenital dislocation of the hips, joint laxity and contractures are common features. Respiratory failure is unusual and less frequent than in nemaline myopathy. Progression, if it occurs, is slow. The serum creatine kinase is usually normal and EMG may be normal or show features of primary muscle disease.

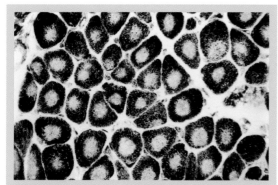

Figure 11.2 Central core disease. NADH-TR stain.

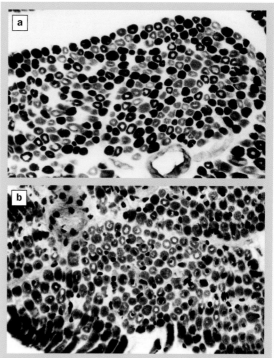

Figure 11.3 Myotubular/centronuclear myopathy. (a) ATPase (pH 9.4); (b) H&E.

There is a complex association with malignant hyperthermia. About one-third of patients with CCD are MH susceptible. Conversely, most patients with MH have normal muscle histology. Unlike porcine MH, human MH shows genetic heterogeneity; some cases have mutations in the ryanodine receptor gene on chromosome 19, some are linked to the sodium channel gene on chromosome 17, but many others do not show linkage to either of these loci. CCD is usually inherited as an autosomal dominant, although sporadic cases have been reported – the significance of this awaits identification of the genetic basis. It is clear that at least some forms of CCD are allelic to MH.

The pathognomonic histological feature consists of centrally, or eccentrically, located cores (Figure 11.2), best seen using the NADH-tetrazolium reductase reaction, which run the length of affected fibres. A common additional feature is type I fibre predominance.

Mini(multi)core disease

This rare condition is defined by the presence of multiple cores, devoid of mitochondria, which unlike those in central core disease only run for short lengths along muscle fibres. The terms multi-core and mini-core have been used interchangeably.

It is usually a relatively mild condition presenting with generalised weakness in early infancy and subsequently with little or no progression. As in nemaline myopathy diaphragmatic weakness and respiratory failure can occur, and skeletal abnormalities are common. Rarely, the extraocular muscles are involved. The serum creatine kinase is normal and EMG shows features of primary muscle disease.

Sporadic cases and autosomal recessive and dominant inheritance have been reported, implying genetic heterogeneity. No genes, or even linkage to a specific chromosome, have yet been described.

Myotubular (centronuclear) myopathy

The names myotubular and centronuclear myopathy have been used interchangeably in the literature. The term myotubular myopathy was proposed because it was thought that the abnormal fibres (Figure 11.3), with central nuclei, resembled myotubes and that the basis of the condition might be arrested maturation. There is no certain evidence for this and there are differences between the abnormal fibres seen in this condition and myotubes. Current convention is to call the severe X-linked form myotubular myopathy, and to use the term centronuclear myopathy for the milder autosomal forms.

The cause of the severe X-linked form is a mutation in the myotubularin gene (*MTMX*) at Xq28. This form is clinically much more homogeneous than the autosomal forms. There is often a history of miscarriages and neonatal male deaths. Those males born alive have severe weakness and respiratory insufficiency and most die in early infancy.

Autosomal forms (both dominant and recessive), for which no genes have yet been identified, are of lesser severity. Onset is usually in infancy or early childhood, rarely in early adult life. Weakness is predominantly proximal and some have facial weakness, ptosis and external ophthalmoplegia. Progression is usually slow or absent.

In all forms the serum creatine kinase is typically normal and EMG shows non-specific myopathic features.

Congenital fibre-type disproportion (CFTD)

The pathological characteristic of this condition is easily defined; there is disproportion between the sizes of type I and type II muscle fibres. Whereas they are normally approximately equal in size, in this condition, due to type II fibre hypertrophy, the difference exceeds 25%. However, there is increasing evidence that this is not a single clinical entity but rather is a heterogeneous syndrome, in which this particular histological pattern may be caused not only by primary muscle disease but also by neurogenic disorders. The phenotype that has most frequently been described in the literature, under the title CFTD, is that of a relatively benign condition.

The "typical" presentation is as a floppy infant. Contractures and congenital dislocation of the hip are common. There is a wide range of severity but marked weakness is uncommon. There is no further progression, and indeed often improvement, after two years of age. Sporadic and autosomal recessive and dominant patterns of inheritance have been reported.

In summary, CFTD is something of a rag-bag diagnosis. There is a mild congenital myopathy (presenting as the so-called floppy baby syndrome) which is associated with the stated histological appearance. It is typically non-progressive, and there may even be improvement after the age of two years. But in addition the same histological appearance may be seen in a number of other conditions, both myopathic and neurogenic, including type I spinal muscular atrophy (Werdnig-Hoffman disease).

Other ultrastructural myopathies

The literature contains many reports, often of single cases, of childhood-onset myopathies which often lack specific clinical features but which are characterised by a disturbance of muscle ultrastructure, reflected in the names given to them; cytoplasmic body myopathy, hyaline body myopathy, zebra body myopathy, fingerprint myopathy, sarcotubular myopathy, reducing body myopathy, tubular aggregate myopathy, desmin storage myopathy, cap disease. Many of these changes are likely to be epiphenomena of the basic, currently unknown, disease process. In other childhood neuromuscular disorders the biopsy shows minor, non-specific changes, to which the term minimal change myopathy has been applied.

Selected further reading

Nemaline myopathy
Nowak KJ, Wattanasirichaigoon D, Goebel HH et al. Mutations in the skeletal muscle alpha-actin gene in patients with actin myopathy and nemaline myopathy. *Nat Genet* 1999; 23: 208–212.
Pelin K, Hilpela P, Donner K et al. Mutations in the nebulin gene associated with autosomal recessive nemaline myopathy. *Proc Natl Acad Sci* 1999; 96: 2305–2310.
Wallgren-Pettersson C, Pelin K et al. Clinical and genetic heterogeneity in autosomal recessive Nemaline myopathy. *Neuromusc Dis* 1999; 9: 564–572.

Central core disease
Bushby M, Squier M. Central core disease. In: Emery AEH (ed). *Neuromuscular Disorders: Clinical and molecular genetics.* Chichester: John Wiley & Sons, 1998: 277–288.

Myotubular (centronuclear) myopathy
Tanner SM, Schneider V, Thomas NST et al. Characterization of 34 novel and six known MTM1 gene mutations in 47 unrelated X-linked myotubular myopathy patients. *Neuromusc Dis* 1999; 9: 41–49.
Wallgren-Pettersson C. 58th ENMC Workshop: Myotubular Myopathy. *Neuromusc Dis* 1998; 8: 521–525.

chapter 12

Neuromuscular junction disorders

Although the neuromuscular junction disorders are not strictly speaking myopathies, they do form an important part of the differential diagnosis of the myopathies. In this chapter we shall therefore present a brief account of myasthenia gravis and related conditions, their diagnosis and treatment.

The neuromuscular junction

Motor nerve action potentials (APs) travel down myelinated fibres by saltatory conduction, with influxing sodium ions creating the local negative potential difference at the nodes of Ranvier. Activation of voltage gated potassium channels lead to an efflux of potassium ions which terminates the local action potential. When the AP reaches the presynaptic membrane of the neuromuscular junction (NMJ), depolarisation causes local influx of calcium ions through voltage gated calcium channels (VGCCs) into the nerve terminal (Figure 12.1). This in turn leads to acetylcholine (ACh) containing vesicles moving towards and fusing with the presynaptic membrane of the neuromuscular junction and results in release of ACh into the synaptic space. The ACh binds to acetylcholine receptors (AChRs) on the post-synaptic membrane which then open to allow cationic influx and ultimately this leads to muscle contraction. The nerve is protected by the blood-nerve barrier except at the nerve terminal making the NMJ a more accessible target than the more proximal part of the nerve for immune-mediated attack. It is clear that disruption anywhere along this pathway can result in dysfunction of neuromuscular transmission.

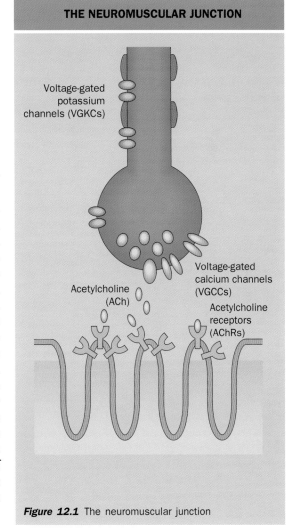

THE NEUROMUSCULAR JUNCTION

Figure 12.1 The neuromuscular junction

Myasthenia gravis

Myasthenia gravis (MG) is an antibody-mediated disorder directed against the postsynaptic NMJ. It affects all races and can occur at any age.

Clinical picture

Patients typically present with fatigable muscle weakness of skeletal muscle. The ocular muscles are usually involved early on and may be solely involved in

Table 12.1 *Subtypes of autoimmune myasthenia gravis*

	Early onset	Thymoma	Late onset	Ocular
Thymic pathology	Hyperplasia	Cortical thymoma	Atrophy	Atrophy
Age of onset	<40 years	Any	>40 years	Any
Sex ratio (F:M)	4:1	1:1	1:2	1:1
Response to thymectomy	Good	Poor	Poor	
Anti-AChR titre	+++	++	0,+	0,+
Frequency	30–40%	10%	30–40%	10–25%

10–25% of cases. Weakness of the limbs including proximal muscles, elbow extension and finger extension is common. Facial and trunk involvement can also occur, respiratory muscle and bulbar involvement can be potentially life threatening. Tendon reflexes are well retained. Patients who develop MG are at greater risk of other autoimmune disorders especially thyroid disease and have a higher rate of other autoantibodies. Eight percent of babies born to mothers with MG have transient neonatal MG due to placental transfer of AChR antibodies. Recent prevalence figures of 1:7,000 and an annual incidence of 1:100,000 have been reported. It is common in young females (who often have thymic hyperplasia and in caucasians an association with HLA B8 and DR3), and also in older males (who show thymic atrophy). It is probably underdiagnosed in this latter group. MG can be divided into subgroups depending on the antibody state, thymus pathology, age of onset and whether generalised or ocular (Table 12.1). This division is relevant to the treatment response. MG may remit temporarily early on but this is seldom permanent and life-long therapy is usually required.

Aetiology
Antibodies to the nicotinic AChR on the NMJ are detectable by radioimmunoprecipitation assay (RIA) in 85% of those with generalised disease and 55% of those with isolated ocular MG. Loss of functional AChRs results: (1) from cross-linking of adjacent AChRs by the antibodies leading to downregulation of AChRs; (2) from compliment mediated lysis of the postsynaptic membrane; and possibly (3) from direct blockade of AChRs. In the patients who are 'seronegative' for anti-AChR antibodies, there appear to be antibodies to a muscle membrane target other than the AChR, that may lead to AChR inactivation through an intracellular pathway. Recently, antibodies against a muscle-specific kinase (MuSK) have been identified in a

number of AChR seronegative patients with generalized MG. In addition some seronegative patients have low titres of antibodies against the epsilon subunit of the AChR (which is present in adult muscle but very little is found in the standard homogenate used in the RIA to detect AChR antibodies). These can be detected however if adult type AChR is added to the assay antigen. The titre of the anti-AChR antibodies correlate only weakly with severity of disease across a population of patients. In an individual patient, however, longitudinal titres follow the disease course more accurately.

The thymus gland is thought to play an important role in the pathogenesis of MG. The normal thymus is a source of AChR – detectable in thymic myoid cells and subunits in thymic epithelial cells – and in addition expression is upregulated in some thymomas. The thymus is also thought to be involved in deleting self-antigen specific T cell clones and therefore any disruption of function could allow escape of auto-reactive T cells. Indeed in MG the thymus is enriched for AChR-reactive T cells and in those with associated thymic hyperplasia, is an anti-AChR antibody-producing site.

Diagnosis
Diagnosis is made by the typical clinical picture, the presence of anti-AChR antibodies and the electrophysiological findings of increased decrement at 3 Hz stimulation and increased jitter and blocking on single fibre EMG. An edrophonium test (Tensilon) test is rarely necessary nowadays with the availability of the other tests although a positive response to oral anticholinesterases such as pyridostigmine is usual. A range of skeletal muscle antibodies to antigens such as α-actin, myosin and titin are often found in those patients with thymoma. The presence of such antibodies is not in itself, however, diagnostic of a thymoma.

Newly diagnosed patients with MG should undergo CT scanning of the chest, seeking to exclude thymoma,

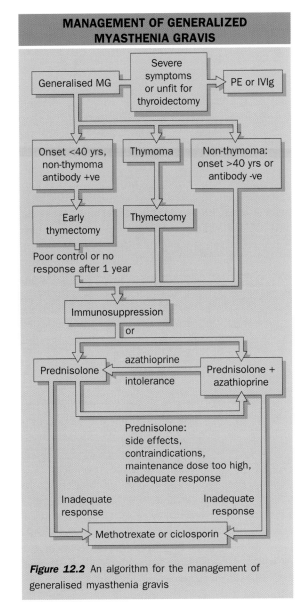

Figure 12.2 An algorithm for the management of generalised myasthenia gravis

and looking for evidence of thymic hyperplasia in younger patients.

Treatment (Figure 12.2)

The first line of treatment is with anticholinesterases (usually pyridostigmine). Thymectomy is indicated for thymoma as long as the patient is fit for general anaesthetic. If there is local invasion of mediastinal tissues or the pleura are breached during surgery, radiotherapy is indicated. If significant symptoms persist despite anticholinesterases, immunosuppression is indicated. In the absence of thymoma, thymectomy should be confined to seropositive cases with early onset age of

onset (<40 years). Twenty-five percent can expect remission and 50% improvement over the next 2–3 years. Prednisolone should be given as a slowly increasing regime and continued on an alternate day dosage until remission occurs. Initiation of corticosteroids can be associated with a temporary deterioration in symptoms and it is therefore advisable to start such treatment as an in-patient unless the patient has ocular or mild generalised MG. At remission the anticholinesterases can be withdrawn and the prednisolone slowly reduced to the minimum required to control symptoms. The addition of azathioprine in generalised MG reduces the maintenance dose of prednisolone. Rarely are other immunosuppressive treatments needed. Plasma exchange (PE) or intravenous immunoglobulin therapy (IVIG) are useful as temporary fast-acting treatments when symptoms are severe. Details of the drugs used are given in Chapter 3.

Lambert–Eaton myasthenic syndrome

The Lambert-Eaton myasthenic syndrome (LEMS) is an autoimmune disorder of the presynaptic NMJ. Sixty percent of patients have a smoking associated small cell lung cancer (SCLC). In non-cancer cases, the disorder can occur from adolescence to extreme old age.

Clinical picture

Patients present in a similar way to those with MG and indeed may be misdiagnosed especially because LEMS is far less common. Proximal muscle weakness often affecting the lower limbs is common. Tendon reflexes tend to be depressed and post-tetanic potentiation may be demonstrable clinically as an increase in the reflexes after maximal voluntary contraction of the relevant muscle. Autonomic symptoms such as dry mouth, constipation and impotence are common but must be actively asked about since they are rarely spontaneously volunteered. A predisposition to other autoimmune diseases and to developing autoantibodies generally is seen in LEMS patients.

Aetiology

Antibodies to the P/Q type voltage gated calcium channels (VGCCs) at motor nerve terminals, on which acetylcholine release depends, are detectable by RIA in 95% of patients. Binding leads to a reduction in quantal release of ACh generated by the motor nerve impulse. The association with small cell lung cancer (SCLC) is interesting since this tumour is thought to originate from neural crest cells and SCLC cell lines express VGCCs. It is suggested that the SCLC triggers an antibody response to its VGCCs, which in turn cross-react with VGCCs on the NMJ to cause LEMS. Indeed macrophage infiltration within SCLC is greater when LEMS is associated. In LEMS with and without SCLC there is an increased frequency of HLA-B8, HLA-DR3 and Ig heavy chain markers but not in those with SCLC alone. This suggests they may be an immune predisposition to developing paraneoplastic LEMS as well as LEMS not associated with malignancy. Even in paraneoplastic LEMS, the responsible tumour may not be evident radiologically for up to five years after the onset of the neurological syndrome. It is therefore recommended that those with a smoking history undergo annual CT scanning of the chest for 5 years after the diagnosis of LEMS is made.

Diagnosis

Increased decrement on repetitive stimulation, and jitter and blocking on single fibre EMG occur as in MG. However, in contrast to MG, the size of the compound muscle action potentials (CMAPs) is reduced, and typically increases by greater than 100% after high frequency nerve stimulation or, easier to tolerate, maximal voluntary contraction. Antibodies to VGCCs are usually detectable.

Treatment

The neuronal potassium channel blocker 3,4–diaminopyridine (3,4–DAP; Chapter 3) and to a lesser extent pyridostigmine often give good symptomatic control (Figure 12.3). They may be used together with added effect. The presence of malignancy is a relative contraindication to immunosuppression. This may be particularly so with LEMS in which there is some evidence that the autoantibodies may themselves suppress tumour growth. However the severity of the syndrome sometimes over-rides this principle. Treatment of the tumour can lead to resolution of the LEMS. Plasma exchange and IVIG can be useful to treat severe symptoms although the effect wears off after a few weeks and some patients need repeated courses.

Acquired neuromyotonia (Isaac's syndrome)

Neuromyotonia is a rare disorder, with a probable autoimmune aetiology, affecting the peripheral motor

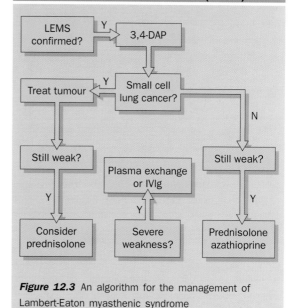

Figure 12.3 An algorithm for the management of Lambert-Eaton myasthenic syndrome

nerves and motor nerve terminals. It has been reported from adolescence onwards.

Clinical features

Acquired neuromyotonia is a syndrome in which patients present with muscle cramps, widespread muscle twitching (visible undulating 'myokymia') which can be triggered by voluntary muscle contraction, and sometimes muscle hypertrophy, stiffness, pseudomyotonia, mild weakness, excess sweating and paraesthesia. Rarely central symptoms such as insomnia and hallucinations occur. Neuromyotonia may be associated with peripheral neuropathies, thymoma (in about 20% of cases), MG and lung carcinoma (three reported cases). The presence of oligoclonal bands in the CSF has been reported in some patients. Remission may occur spontaneously.

Aetiology

Antibodies directed against voltage gated potassium channels (VGKCs) and causing peripheral nerve hyper-excitability would make a good theoretical pathological candidate in this condition and are detectable in 50% of cases with a RIA using α-dendrotoxin. This toxin does not however bind all VGKC and therefore not all anti-VGKC antibodies would be detected by this assay. The increased motor nerve excitability leads to spontaneous firing and prolonged discharges after voluntary activation. It can be explained by the antibodies reducing the function of VGKCs that normally terminate the local action potential by repolarisation. The positive response to plasma exchange in such patients further supports an autoimmune aetiology. In addition D-penicillamine, which is well recognised as a causal factor in precipitating autoimmune diseases such as MG (associated with the HLA Bw35 and DR1 haplotypes) and systemic lupus erythematosus, has been reported to induce neuromyotonia.

Diagnosis

EMG shows typical doublet, triplet and multiple single unit discharges of high intraburst frequency (Figure 12.4). The bursts occur irregularly. The abnormality continues during sleep and general anaesthesia and also distal to peripheral nerve block, but not after local curare, suggesting that the abnormality arises from increased excitability of distal motor nerves (motor nerve terminus as well as the nodes of Ranvier). Creatine kinase is often raised but does not reflect any primary muscle disease.

Treatment

Carbamazepine and phenytoin can control symptoms in some patients. Plasma exchange and immunosuppression may be necessary in others.

Congenital myasthenic syndromes

Congenital myasthenic syndromes (CMS) are a rare heterogeneous group of inherited disorders affecting neuromuscular transmission. They can be divided into three categories depending on the location of the defect: postsynaptic (acetylcholine receptor deficiency – the most common CMS in the UK, slow-channel syndrome, low affinity fast channel syndrome), synaptic (acetylcholinesterase deficiency), or presynaptic (e.g. familial infantile myasthenia).

Clinical features

Onset is usually in the neonatal period or in infancy except in the slow channel syndrome, which may not present until adulthood. As with MG any skeletal muscle can be affected and ocular muscles are

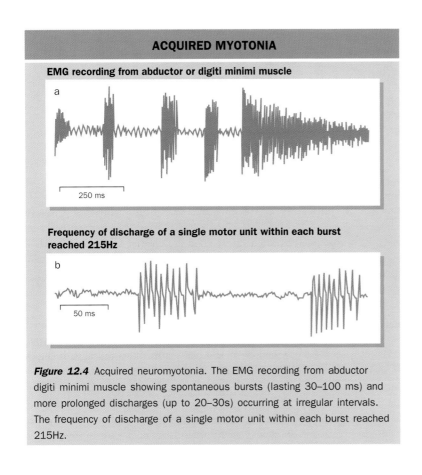

ACQUIRED MYOTONIA

EMG recording from abductor or digiti minimi muscle

a

250 ms

Frequency of discharge of a single motor unit within each burst reached 215Hz

b

50 ms

Figure 12.4 Acquired neuromyotonia. The EMG recording from abductor digiti minimi muscle showing spontaneous bursts (lasting 30–100 ms) and more prolonged discharges (up to 20–30s) occurring at irregular intervals. The frequency of discharge of a single motor unit within each burst reached 215Hz.

Table 12.2 *Genetic basis of congenital myasthenic syndromes*

Syndrome	Genetic basis
Anticholinesterase deficiency	11 mutations (single amino acid substitutions, deletions, insertions) in *ColQ* gene (attaches acetylcholinesterase to basal lamina)
Slow channel syndrome	>15 nucleotide missense mutations across all four subunits of adult type AChR
AChR deficiency	>40 mutations (insertions, deletions, splice site and missense mutations, promotor region mutations); majority in ε subunit
Low-affinity fast channel	Three mutations; two missense and one short duplication in α and ε subunits

AChR, acetylcholine receptor

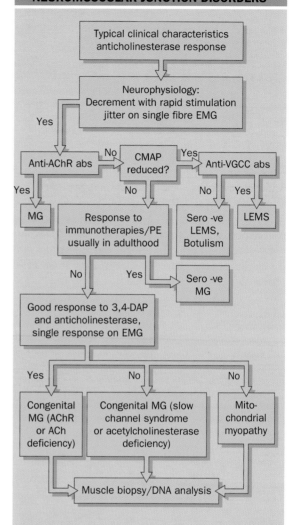

Figure 12.5 An approach to the differential diagnosis of neuromuscular junction disorders

commonly involved. The muscle weakness can be severe and affect respiratory and bulbar muscles, and in familial infantile myasthenia, tends to improve with age. A progressive syndrome of limb girdle weakness often with involvement of the finger extensors and without ocular weakness is common in the slow channel syndrome.

Aetiology

Genetic mutations have been identified for the synaptic (acetylcholinesterase) and post-synaptic (AChR) congenital myasthenic syndromes (Table 12.2). The non-immune aetiology is supported by the lack of specific autoantibodies directed against the NMJ and the lack of response to immune therapies.

Diagnosis

The typical neurophysiological features of impaired neuromuscular transmission are found on conventional neurophysiological assessment. Occasionally difficulties arise differentiating between young onset antibody negative MG and CMS. A family history, consanguinity of the parents or the discovery of affected relatives when examined in the clinic, supports the diagnosis. A lack of response to immune therapies such as plasma exchange can be helpful. Intercostal muscle biopsy for morphological, biochemical and electrophysiological studies of the NMJ, and DNA analysis may be performed. Where a congenital myasthenic syndrome is

suspected, formal evaluation of neuromuscular transmission by intracellular recording from muscle end plates is required. Because whole muscle fibres are required this usually requires biopsy from the motor end plates of short muscle fibres, and the intercostal muscles are favoured. Recordings are then made in vitro. A repetitive response to single nerve stimulation and prolongation of the miniature end plate potential (MEPP) decay phase on muscle biopsy is seen with acetylcholinesterase deficiency and the slow channel syndrome and there are other characteristic findings.

Table 12.3 *Aetiology of neuromuscular junction disorders*

Myasthenia gravis	Lambert–Eaton myasthenic syndrome	Neuromyotonia	Congenital myasthenic syndromes
Postsynaptic	Presynaptic	Presynaptic (nerve and terminal)	Presynaptic, synaptic, postsynaptic
Anti-acetylcholine receptor antibodies	Anti-voltage gated calcium channel antibodies	Anti-voltage gated potassium channel antibodies	No antibodies

Treatment

Anticholinesterases and 3,4–diaminopyridine are helpful except in acetylcholinesterase deficiency and the slow channel syndrome in which symptoms can be exacerbated. Ephedrine, quinine sulphate and fluoxetine have been reported to be helpful in patients with the slow channel syndrome.

A flow diagram that may assist in the differential diagnosis of the neuromuscular junction disorders is given in Figure 12.5 and their aetiology in Table 12.3.

Suggested further reading

Beeson D, Jacobson L, Newsom-Davis J, Vincent A. A transfected human muscle cell line expressing the adult subtype of the human muscle acetylcholine receptor for diagnostic assays in myasthenia gravis. *Neurology* 1996; 47: 1552–1555.

Engel AG, Ohno K, Sine SM. Congenital myasthenic syndromes: recent advances. *Arch Neurol* 1999; 56:163–167.

Maddison P, Newsom-Davis J, Mills KR, Souhami RL. Favourable prognosis in Lambert-Eaton myasthenic syndrome and small-cell lung carcinoma. *Lancet* 1999; 353:117–118.

Palace J, Newsom-Davis J, Lecky B and the Myasthenia Gravis Study Group. A randomised double-blind trial of prednisolone alone or with azathioprine in myasthenia gravis. *Neurology* 1998; 50:1778–1783.

Robertson NP, Deans J, Compston DA. Myasthenia gravis: a population based epidemiological study in Cambridgeshire, England. *J Neurol Neurosurg Psychiatry* 1998; 65:492–498.

Sanders DB. Lambert-Eaton myasthenic syndrome: clinical diagnosis, immune-mediated mechanisms, and update on therapies. *Ann Neurol* 1995; 37(Suppl 1): S63–S73.

Vincent A, Jacobson L, Plested CP et al. Antibodies affecting ion channel function in acquired neuromyotonia, in seropositive and seronegative myasthenia gravis, and in antibody-mediated arthrogryposis multiplex congenita. *Ann NY Acad Sci* 1998; 841: 482–496.

Index

Page numbers in *italics* indicate figures or tables.

bacteria, causing myositis 93
Becker muscular dystrophy (BMD) 59–60
    cardiac involvement 53, *53*, 64, 67
    clinical features 10, 64
    diagnosis 27, *60*, 65–6
    female carriers 60
        manifesting 60, 64, 68
    genetic counselling 66
    genetics and pathophysiology 61, 62
    management 66–7
    muscle biopsy 35–6, *36*, 65–6, *65*
Becker's myotonia congenita 97, 99
    clinical features 98–9
    pathophysiology and genetics 105–6, *105*
    treatment 100
bed rest, adverse effects 54, 63
benzodiazepines 52
β-oxidation defects 109–10, 119–22, *121*
    biochemistry 119, *120*
    clinical features 119–22
    investigations 122
    management 122
Bethlem myopathy 74–5
bicycle exercise test, aerobic 28, 32
biochemistry 26–33
bioenergetics, muscle *28*, 29–31
blocking phenomenon 24–5
blood disorders 11
blood tests 26–8
bone disease, metabolic 145
bowel pseudo-obstruction 10–11
bradyarrhythmias *53*
branching enzyme *29*, 126
    deficiency 9, 136
Brody's syndrome 5, 15

caffeine contracture test 104
calcifications, subcutaneous 88
calcium channelopathies 97, *97*
    pathophysiology and genetics 106, *106*
calcium channels
    skeletal muscle 106, *106*
    voltage-gated (VGCCs) 155, 157–8
calf pseudohypertrophy 63, *63*, 99
calpain-3 mutations 67, *68*
candidate genes 38
carbohydrate
    load, in periodic paralysis 100, 101–2
    metabolism, disorders of 125–37
cardiac disease
    assessment 9, *9*, 15

    in Becker muscular dystrophy 53, *53*, 64, 67
    in debrancher enzyme deficiency 133
    in Duchenne muscular dystrophy 53, *53*, 64, 67
    in Emery–Dreifuss dystrophy 53, *53*, 73–4
    in inflammatory myopathies *53*, 88
    investigations 39
    management 53–4
    in myotonic dystrophy 53, *53*, 76–7, 79
    patterns 53–4, *53*
cardiomyopathy 9, *9*, 53, *53*
    in β-oxidation defects 119
    dilated 53–4, 64–5
    in Emery–Dreifuss dystrophy 74
    in glycogenolytic/glycolytic disorders 136–7
    in mitochondrial myopathies 115
cardiorespiratory function *50*
carnitine 119, *120*
    deficiency 120, *121*, 122
    supplements 122
carnitine palmitoyl transferase (CPT) deficiency 119,
        120–1, *121*
    biochemistry 119, *120*
    investigations 37–8, 122
cataracts, in myotonic dystrophy 77, 79
caveolin-3 mutations 67, *68*
cell surface proteins 62, *62*
central core disease (CCD) 103, 151–2, *152*
central nervous system (CNS) involvement 9–10, *9*, 15
    in congenital muscular dystrophy 80, *81*
    in mitochondrial myopathies 9–10, *9*, 113, *114*, 115
    in myotonic dystrophy 10, 77
centronuclear myopathy 152–3, *152*
channelopathies 97–107, *97*
    investigations *20*, 21
    myotonias 98–100
    pathophysiology and genetics 104–6
    therapy 43–4, *43*
    see also malignant hyperthermia; periodic paralyses
childhood, specific features of 15
chlorambucil 95
chloride channelopathies 97, 99
    pathophysiology and genetics 105–6, *105*
    see also Becker's myotonia congenita; myotonia
        congenita; Thomsen's disease
chloroquine 141
cholesterol-lowering agents 140
cholinesterase (ChE) 44
chondrodysplastic myotonia 99
chronic fatigue syndrome 4
chronic progressive external ophthalmoplegia (CPEO)
        113–14